Relieve your pain and allow
with the miraculo

BOWEN THERAPY

Tom Bowen's gift to the world

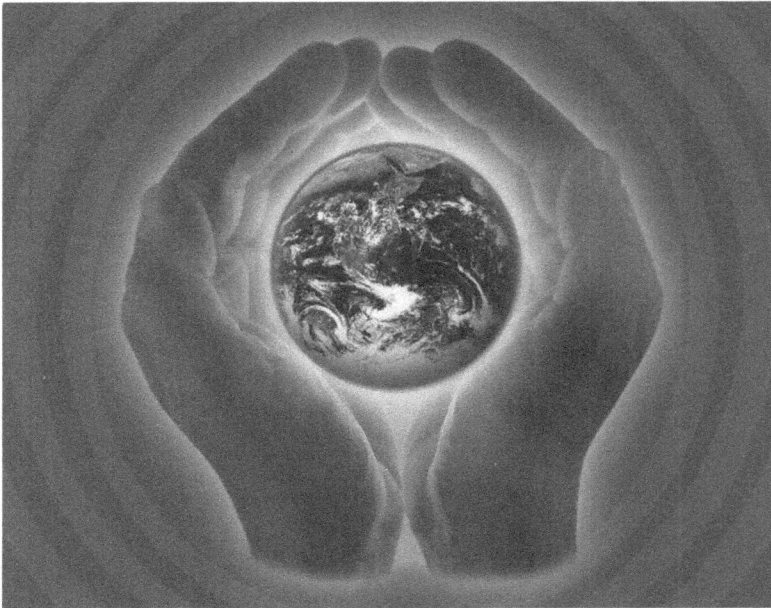

Frank Navratil, BSc. N.D.

The information in this book is for educational purposes only. It is not intended for use in practice except by qualified accredited practitioners who have undergone training in the Bowen method. The material is based on the best available research and study by the author at the time of printing and many years experience in Bowen Therapy. The author and publisher are not responsible for any unauthorized use of this method or for any errors in the text or diagrams in this book.

Published by Frank Navratil BSc. N.D.
Return to Health Books
Purkynova 1246/9
Ricany
Czech Republic
Second Edition
© 2014 Frank Navratil
ISBN 978-80-88022-04-6

TOUCH

Beneath my skin I hide within

and wait

for your current to flow through

for in me is an endless river

of feeling

to the surface I call

to where

you will place an open hand

there

where a big heart will beat

only in touch

can mind, body and soul meet

Helena Dostálová and Frank Navratil

Contents

Acknowledgements

As always, I would like to thank my mother Ludmila Navratil, who died from cancer many years ago. Her inspiration and courage is always with me and has inspired me to pursue alternative medicine and to learn about natural methods that allow the body to heal itself.

I would like to thank the thousands of my patients for their belief and support because thanks to them I was able to learn much about Bowen Therapy. They have allowed me to gather an abundance of research material so that I could write and share what I had learned.

Many thanks to all the accredited Bowen Therapy students who have taken my courses. They will be the new generation and will continue the pioneering work that Tom Bowen began.

Thanks again to Hanka Kopecká for her love, patience and support while I labored at the time-consuming task of writing this book.

I would like to thank Thomas Ambrose Bowen, even though I never knew him, his spirit and energy are with all those who have chosen to follow in his footsteps.

I would also like to thank all of my devoted readers, who have stayed with me through my pursuits to learn, study, teach and write about the value of natural medicine. Together we will make a change in this world.

Finally, for those who "by coincidence" have come face to face with natural medicine and Bowen Therapy for the first time, I thank you for taking the time to learn about this wonderful method and I sincerely hope that it can improve your body's ability to heal itself by natural means.

Preface

As the fog lifts, uncover the secrets of Bowen Therapy

It was not a coincidence that I came to learn about the method of Bowen Therapy, just as it was not a coincidence that I was inspired to move to Australia from Canada, nor to take what I had learned to the Czech Republic. As each one of us has a mission in this life, I believe that mine is to help people to come to a greater awareness of how natural methods can provide healing assistance.

It is also not a coincidence that you have decided to read this book. There is a multitude of events that have led you to opening its cover just as there have been an incomprehensible series of events that have preceded my writing of it. Perhaps you are burdened with back or neck pain that just doesn't seem to go away or perhaps you suffer from migraine headaches. Perhaps you are searching for an alternative method to assist your health problems other than those used in modern medicine. Maybe you are tired of taking drugs and painkillers and would just like to find a natural way to deal with your chronic conditions. Whatever the reason you have chosen to read this book, I am sure it will enlighten you to a natural method that is revolutionizing health care around the world.

I believe that we learn from encountering others around us as well as from those from the past, but I also believe that when we are touched or inspired by them even after their death, their energy and spirit stays with us.

What we do with these encounters or so-called coincidences is entirely up to us. They can drift by us just as passing mist on a foggy day or they can adhere, permeate the inner reaches of our soul and shape and form our destiny.

Inspiration is a strong mediator of change. It comes from encounters with events and from people around us that we can identify with or that are close to us. When we are inspired we have the ability to make a change. Again that change can be a fleeting one as that passing mist on a foggy day or a permanent one that has the ability to shape and change our life in ways that we have never dreamt possible.

Many years ago I too found myself amidst the fog and encountered a passing mist and chose not to ignore it but to follow its course. It came in the form of a suggestion while living in Australia by an acquaintance to enroll in learning a miraculous technique, called Bowen Therapy. One encounters many natural healing methods throughout life but this method was particularly close to me right from the beginning. It was not a fleeting mist that just passes by. It inspired me to not only learn and study the Bowen method but to practice and eventually teach and pass on my experiences to others.

The Bowen method has been responsible for thousands of cases around the world for what modern medicine calls miracles. As mysterious as its founder, Tom Bowen, its success has puzzled even the greatest doctors of our time. What this really means is that we still know very little about the human body and how it works. It is true that we have mountains of books on anatomy and physiology and knowledge and theories of how our body systems interact together but I believe that we have only uncovered the tip of the iceberg of what we know about our health. The Bowen method seems to go beyond the physical understanding that modern medicine has today.

With modern society have come modern health problems. Back and neck pain is one of the most common complaints in the world today. Every other person complains about being under intense stress. Chronic fatigue is showing up with alarming rates. Migraine headaches are on the rise. What is happening to our body? It seems that it is losing its natural balance and we require this balance to maintain all our body functions.

The sad thing is that most of us tend to treat our health problems with some sort of chemical drug, painkillers for neck and back pain, for headaches and migraines, as well as a host of other drugs that claim to heal our ailing conditions. The reality is they do not cure our conditions but only serve to curb the symptoms temporarily and leave the cause of the disease untreated, not to mention those dangerous side effects.

The core cause of a disease is not an easy task to uncover. Many factors are responsible for diseases and the symptoms that we feel. Unfortunately there is no miracle drug for most of the chronic diseases that we suffer from today. The causes of the health problem have to be tackled holistically, from all angles, which often include nutritional imbalances, psychological causes, lack of exercise, lifestyle habits, levels of stress and amount of water intake. This is the only way that we really can cure the disease at the core level. Bowen Therapy plays an intricate role in balancing energy levels in the body, releasing muscle and nervous tension and revitalizing a congested lymphatic system, often responsible for a variety of pain and inflammation in the body, high anxiety or depression, low immunity or high levels of toxins in the body. In its own wonderful way Bowen acts holistically on all parts of the body, regaining its natural balance. In short, along with proper nutrition and lifestyle habits, it allows favorable conditions that allow the body to heal itself.

Many years of performing Bowen therapy on thousands of patients have convinced me that this gentle non-invasive method has successfully assisted a wide range of health problems ranging from diverse conditions as tinnitus, back pain, cysts, gynecological problems, to migraines, asthma, depression, stress and countless others. It has also been responsible in preventing many unnecessary surgical operations.

I believe that Bowen therapy is one of the greatest discoveries of modern health. I sincerely hope that this opportunity to learn about it does not pass you by as a fleeting whisp of fog but provides direction, inspiration, solution to your health problems and above all change in your views on natural medicine.

I am ever optimistic that as the fog lifts and as you gain more knowledge about the needs of your individual body it will become more and more clear what you must do to achieve optimum health.

Frank Navratil BSc. N.D.

BOWEN THERAPY

Tom Bowen's gift to the world

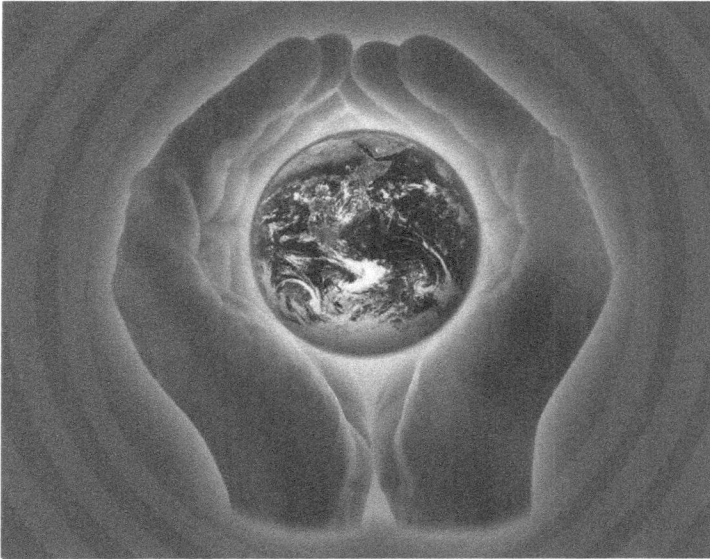

Introduction:

A unique, gentle and effective method that allows the body to heal itself

Introduction:

A unique, gentle and effective method that allows the body to heal itself

Welcome to my book about the wonderful method of Bowen therapy, a natural non-invasive healing method that is capturing the hearts of health care professionals and healers around the world. This book is designed as a resource for patients who are interested in or undergoing Bowen therapy or for those who would simply like to learn more about this intriguing method, which is used by doctors, healers, accredited massage therapists, physiotherapists, nurses and laypeople, and taught and practiced in well over 25 countries around the world. It is not intended as an instruction manual but as a general overview of how Bowen therapy works, what it is comprised of and the benefits that can be achieved.

The Bowen method is a dynamic technique of muscle and connective tissue release that has started a revolution in health care. It has been used successfully for over 40 years and has helped thousands of patients. It has puzzled therapists and doctors as to how exactly it works and if Tom Bowen was alive today, many who have used his methods would surely like to ask him why his technique works so effectively.

The Bowen method uses only gentle moves but yields outstanding results that even the modern medicine circles have taken notice. Often relief from serious back and neck pain, migraine headaches, frozen shoulder or knee pain is achieved after only a few sessions. There have even been cases where improvement from scoliosis and other curvatures of the spine occurred. The method is also widely used for assisting other health problems such as tinnitus, allergies, asthma, bladder infections, high or low blood pressure, depression and psychological problems, eczema, gallbladder pain, kidney and menstrual conditions. Improvements are often seen in immune function, kidney function, joint mobility and breathing ability as well as assistance in countless other chronic and acute health conditions.

The amazing feature of Bowen therapy is a series of precise, gentle and painless pressure moves, which are applied over clothing, which improve energy flow in the body and aid in self-healing.

If I could describe Bowen therapy in one sentence, I would say that it is not massage, it is not acupressure or acupuncture, nor is it energy healing or reiki, but it embraces some aspects of each of these methods, making it a unique method of its own and often yielding impressive results.

Most important of all, it is safe for everyone from newborns to the elderly. The Bowen method regains the body's state of balance, allows for natural regeneration and releases muscle tension, which are often the result of poor posture, lack of exercise or injury.

Just think of all the abuse we place on our bodies. We sleep on poor mattresses with too many pillows so that the spine and muscles are placed in unnatural positions and are not adequately rested. We don't exercise enough and we often wear poor quality gym shoes that do not cushion our spine. We lift objects without bending our knees, which strains our back and increases the chance of injuries. When we sit in the driving seat we often turn our torso to reach for something in the back, again leading to strains and injuries. Commonly we carry bags on one shoulder further placing strain on one side of the body instead of as the Africans do, carry objects on their heads. Not surprisingly they have a lot less back problems than we do! There are many more other unhealthy activities that our bodies are subjected to and which cause imbalances in posture as well as placing stress on our spine.

As a result of this imbalance our muscles are forced to react in defense by cramping, contracting and trying to compensate which often leads to muscle tightening, pain and greater tension on one side of the body. Often flexibility is then reduced; limbs freeze up and lose their full range of motion. The nervous system can also be drastically affected which can lead to poorly functioning organs, digestive problems and other nerve-related dysfunctions.

Bowen therapy uses positive and negative moves that stimulate and isolate energy flow in specific regions of the body. For example, there are specific series of moves for the kidneys, the lower back, neck and other body areas. Probably the greatest difference between the Bowen method and other body therapies is the Bowen move itself, which you will learn about in a further chapter in this book. Performing all the moves in a specific series provides the best results.

Are you suffering from:

Back or neck pain?

Frequent headaches or migraines?

Chronic fatigue?

Annoying colds or flu?

Stress or depression?

Pre-menstrual syndrome?

Edema or swelling?

Asthma or breathing difficulties?

Skin problems?

Digestive problems?

Arthritis or joint problems?

Frozen shoulder?

If you are, you will most likely benefit from Bowen therapy. As a result of the Bowen method, whatever tension in the body is usually dramatically reduced or completely alleviated. Inflammation is lessened and cysts and edema may even disappear. It seems that the Bowen method stimulates the detoxification organs in the body such as the kidneys, liver and lymphatic system to rid the body of wastes and toxins, thus improving over-all immunity and preventing infections and disease.

For pregnant mothers, the Bowen method is excellent for relieving back pain due to changes in the body.

Although Bowen therapy is not specifically designed to deal with psychological problems, often anxiety, depression and intense stress are improved. Patients report feelings that a burden has been taken off of their backs, they begin to see their problems more clearly and their stressful lives become easier to manage.

Improvement in energy levels and well-being often are cited commonly after a Bowen therapy session and I have seen migraine headaches disappear in intense sufferers for up to six months or more.

This method originating from Australia has been so successful that veterinarians have even used it on horses, dogs and other animals.

The Bowen method brings outstanding results. Not always but in a large proportion of cases. As the world of modern medicine attempts to scientifically decipher these methods developed by the great pioneer of this work, the late Tom Bowen and prove how they work, the thousands of therapists actively using his method around the world are simply satisfied with the fact that is just works and is safe to use for everyone.

Simply stated, Bowen therapy is a unique, gentle and effective method that allows the body to heal itself and in my opinion one the most miraculous discoveries of natural medicine.

BOWEN THERAPY

Tom Bowen's gift to the world

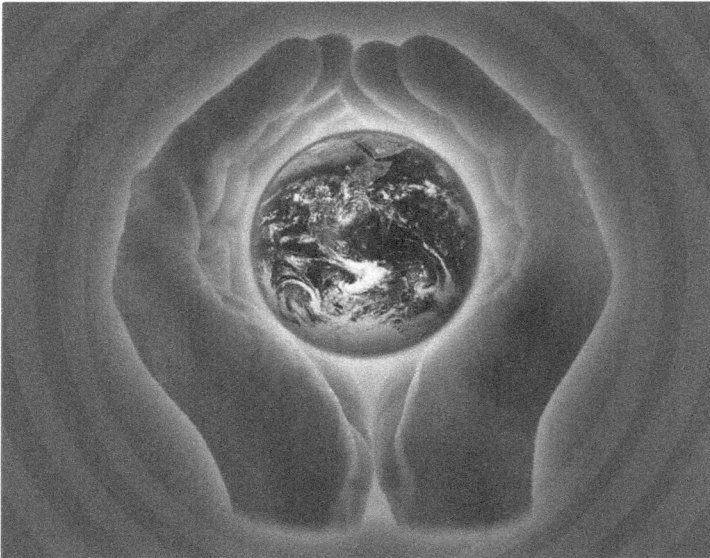

Part 1

Promoting a healing environment

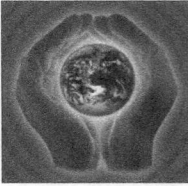

The significance of touch in the body's healing process

A healing environment involves many components and studies have shown that several factors in our environment including color, smells, sound and touch have powerful therapeutic effects. A healing environment often leads to faster recovery from diseases and infection and reduction of pain.

As we perceive our environment through our senses of touch, sight, smell, taste and hearing, information that is relayed to the brain affects both our psychological as well as our physical being.

We require many nutrients for survival including food, water and oxygen but what is often forgotten or taken for granted is our need for touch.

Many scientific studies have clearly demonstrated that babies who do not have contact in the form of touch do not grow normally. It has been shown that touch and massage and other body therapies on infants and toddlers resulted in better sleeping habits, improved asthma in young children and reduced hyperactivity in attention deficit disorder adolescents. Even autistic children have responded favorably to therapies using touch.

In recent times touch in the form of massage therapies has been used to counter a host of conditions from depression, stress, anxiety, anorexia, bulimia, chronic fatigue, dermatitis, low immunity, childhood diabetes, hypertension to migraines, premenstrual symptoms, Alzheimer's disease and cravings for smoking. It seems that many health problems react favorably to touch and we are only starting to understand its affect on the human body. There is even a place for compassionate touch for the terminally ill and cancer patients who have responded positively.

Compassionate touch is a very powerful healing tool which can provide assistance to create an environment favorable for self-healing from neonates to the sick and elderly.

There are many forms of touch from holding a hand, holding an infant, romantic touch, sexual touch, compassionate touch and a variety of body therapies including reflexology, shiatsu, craniosacral therapy, acupressure, kinesiology, and of course Bowen therapy, the subject of this book. All of these body therapies mentioned have healing capabilities in the form of touch and benefit a variety of conditions. Which one do you choose? Again, I believe that your intuition and experience will help you with this and you will decide what method is best for you. I chose the Bowen method among all these that I was presented with. I felt closest to this method and its principles of natural healing. Perhaps by the end of this book you too will be convinced, as I am, that Bowen therapy is the greatest health discovery in modern medicine. Read my real-life case studies at the end of this book to convince yourself.

It seems that Bowen therapy provides a safe and neutral environment for patients to receive the healing effect of touch that is so important for emotional health and self-esteem. Touch seems to be a fundamental component for the development of a healthy human being and lack of touch is known to inhibit the physical and emotional development of children. It seems in normal society as one ages, the power of touch and the comfort of touch has been largely forgotten. Infants usually receive the most touch, which is essential for their survival, but by the time we reach old age, it dwindles to the bare minimum. Perhaps this is one part of the reason for increased incidence of depression in old age, high blood pressure and senility. It is not surprising that interest in body therapies such as massage and the Bowen method have grown incredibly over the last 20 years. More people today engage in regular massage and other body therapies than ever before. Perhaps they are compensating for society's minimum contact in the form of friendly touch.

I believe that the Bowen method is an active form of touch, which not only unlocks physical tensions trapped in muscles and connective tissue but also promotes an essence of calmness and caring for that person which is often lacking in this non-personal world today. I believe it is a beneficial method because it assists the client to feel safe enough to relax and unwind from the deepest parts of the mind and body. This form of touch has the ability to result in emotional release and the feeling of security often brings unresolved psychological problems to the surface.

Many body therapies including forms of massage teach that cancer is a contradiction but I believe that Bowen therapy due to its gentleness is beneficial during the cancer process. It is important during such critical illnesses that both physical and emotional needs are cared for and touch in the form of Bowen therapy is ideal.

We should always remember that touch is the most enduring and closest of human interactions, which begins from our mother's cradling arms around us, through to a hug by our parents, the shaking of hands with a friend, the passionate embrace, to the parting touch when we are dying. Touch provides the assurance that we are alive, that we are cared for and that we are worthwhile of living. Even our life expectancy has shown to be diminished when there is a deprivation of touch, showing us that it really is a human need that we cannot live without. **Have you been touched lately with the Bowen method?**

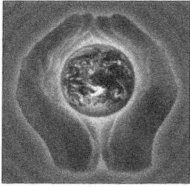

How the body can lose its delicate balance

The terms "homeostasis" or "dynamic equilibrium" are often used to describe a situation where change is constantly occurring but a state of balance is always being achieved. We are in dynamic balance with the world around us. Nature is a complex association of change that is constantly kept in check; our thermostat maintains a comfortable heating level in our homes despite cold air that enters when we open the door. We can say that a state of dynamic balance is a healthy, natural way to be. A healthy dynamic balance can resist dramatic changes that are imposed and quickly make adjustment so that equilibrium is maintained.

Our bodies need to be in a state of balance in order for optimum health to be achieved.

Stresses are often imposed that shift the balance in one direction or the other and in most cases the body can adjust and regain the balance. However if these stresses become more than the body can handle the state of balance begins to break down. This places the body in a vulnerable situation, one where it can no longer keep balance and thus opens the gateway to disease conditions and injuries.

How does the body lose its balance?

Ultimately it comes down to one or more organs or tissues that break down and cannot perform their job very well anymore. It is then difficult to maintain such a delicate balance in the body. Take for example, a common fever. If there is infection or inflammation in the body, the body reacts and raises the temperature to destroy the pathological bacteria or virus. In a relatively healthy body with a relatively healthy immune system the fever lasts only a short time. In a weak body with a poor immune system the fever can last much longer and even reach life-threatening levels. It all comes down to the body's ability to combat stresses and maintain equilibrium.

The same can occur when our bodies are malnourished, when we do not have adequate sleep, when our water intake is low, when we are under intense emotional stress or when we do not exercise. Eventually cells do not receive the nutrients and rest that they require. They begin to weaken and die, this affects the tissues and finally the muscles and organs. Somewhere the state of balance in the body has been altered. What did we say was the result? - a gateway to disease and injuries.

As almost 80 percent of clients that come for Bowen therapy suffer from some sort of back or neck problem, it is useful to look at how the state of delicate balance in the body has been offset to such a level that it becomes very difficult to regain on its own.

Commonly some sort of strain is placed while lifting or turning or moving. Now the muscles of the body are designed to hold that skeleton in place and in order to do that job they have to be exercised. Muscles that are not exercised lose their strength, deteriorate, and begin to atrophy. They become less efficient at supporting our bones and spine and make it easier for injury to occur. Not to mention our ligaments, which lose flexibility if not stretched and they too become vulnerable to injury. So, we cannot expect an unexercised and inflexible body to react to physical activities such as lifting, turning or moving as well as one that is fine-tuned and in balance. One of the keys to preventative health is that one must exercise regularly to maintain balance in the body. This means throughout life and even well into old age.

Our emotional state of health plays a large role in our physical health. If we are under emotional stress our body organs do not function smoothly, our digestive processes are diminished and our nutritional needs are often increased. This can place the body in a deficit situation or in a state of imbalance. It is therefore important to resolve inner conflicts, to rid yourself of negative emotions that just may be preventing your body from regaining its ability to heal itself.

What is the role of Bowen Therapy in the body's delicate balance?

The Bowen method is a natural healing technique that balances energy flow in the body. It follows the basic premise that the body cannot heal itself if it is not in balance. Energy flow is critical for the body's healing capabilities and for all the essential life processes. The Bowen method assists in achieving dynamic equilibrium in the body.

What are the rewards for maintaining our bodies in dynamic equilibrium?

Well to start, we will be able to resist disease more effectively; we will be less prone to injury and better prepared to handle stress. We will feel less tired and have far more energy to do the things that we love to do. A body in dynamic equilibrium is an optimum state of health where the mind, body and spirit are in harmony. When we achieve optimum health we are also able to think clearer, and generally are much more happier. Don't you think that it something that is worth achieving?

It is common for our body to fall prey to imbalances and to lose its state of dynamic equilibrium. The best way to avoid back problems and other health problems is to prevent them from happening in the first place. As we will learn in the next chapter, there are many components that influence our health and well-being, and go far beyond just the physical.

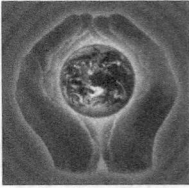

The holistic wheel of health and individual differences

The fact that each one of us is different often makes it very difficult to find a cure for our individual health problems. The causes for each one of them are always different. You may believe that you have tried everything in the book to rid yourself of that back pain or migraine headache but perhaps you have only touched the tip of the iceberg. Holistic health involves an entire spectrum of components that influence our well-being. Getting rid of the cause of pain is not just as simple as popping a pill and waiting for it to go away. You will not permanently cure your disease that way but only temporarily suppress the symptoms. Finding the true core cause of health problems involves an analysis of all the holistic factors

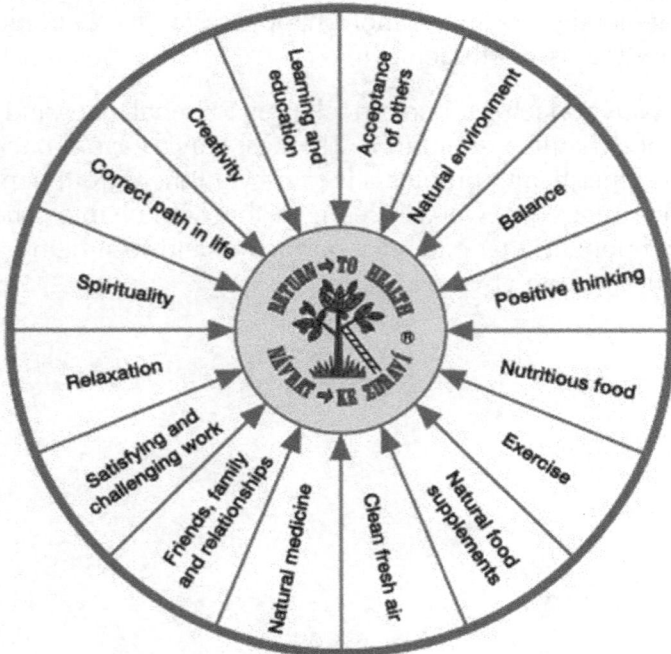

The Holistic Wheel of Health

that influence health. This is the only complete method that takes into consideration our individual differences. I call it the holistic wheel of health. The Bowen Method is one slice of that pie, one segment of that wheel, that component of touch that provides a significant healing hand when we encounter imbalances in the body but there are many others to take into consideration. Ask yourself if any of these other factors could be contributing to your ill health.

Some holistic influences on health include:

Poor Nutrition

I believe that poor nutrition is in some form or another a cause of 90 percent of our health problems today. When I speak to patients about their diet it is not surprising that they are experiencing back pain or the health problems that they have. Remember quality nutrition is essential for all our life processes. Without adequate nutrition our body cannot heal itself or regenerate its tissues. If you are interested in learning more about holistic nutrition please read my book, *The Eye for an Eye Diet.*

Lack of Water

The energy that your life processes require can be quickly depleted when there is insufficient water intake or poor quality of water. Remember, the body is made of over 70 percent water. You need water for numerous reactions and functions in the body. You require water to flush the body and detoxify. Your health, your skin and your mood will all improve with an increase in water intake. If you suffer from back or arthritis problems, migraines, chronic fatigue or other debilitating conditions, ask yourself if you are drinking enough fresh, clean, un-carbonated water. It may be one of the main reasons why you are suffering from disease. As a special consideration for Bowen therapy to be fully effective, it is required that you increase your water intake substantially during treatment.

Lack of Exercise

Most people have a tendency to adopt a sedentary lifestyle. The activity level of our youth fades away and we get bogged down with life's responsibilities such as work and family commitments. The thought of having to exercise after a long workday to many is inconceivable.

Exercise however, is crucial if we want to be free of heart problems, backache, menstrual difficulties, stress, weight problems as well as almost every single disease imaginable. We just can't achieve optimum health if we don't exercise our bodies. There are just so many reasons why exercise is needed. Exercise stimulates our circulation, digestion, absorption, detoxification and regeneration functions, all of which are essential to the efficient operation of the body.

Lack of clean, fresh air and deep breathing

Air contains oxygen and oxygen is one of the life-giving substances that our body needs. Air also contains contaminants due to smog and pollution and that is what we don't need. The decrease in clean, oxygen-rich air that we breathe in contributes to our growing health problems. On top of that, and largely due to stress, we are not breathing properly or deeply enough resulting in low levels of oxygen. Remember, we require oxygen for our metabolism, to burn fats, to produce energy so that all of our essential processes of life can function.

Try to live in areas with little or no pollution and if you can't, get to a park, the mountains or the ocean as often as you can. Many of my patients who have serious degenerative health problems have reported significant improvements when they began to breathe in clean, fresh unpolluted air.

Lack of Relaxation and quality sleep

Every other person that has entered my clinic has reported being under severe stress, experiencing problems sleeping or suffering from pressure in the workplace. Ask yourself if you work too much and if you give yourself at least some time everyday to relax and release stress and care for your well-being. Do not underestimate the effect that stress has on your physical health. Periods of stress often precede many cancers that I have seen as well as back and neck pain, migraines, hormonal problems, heart problems and digestive disturbances. Lack of relaxation will not allow the body to do its best and will slow down the healing process.

Sleep is one of the most important nutrients that our mind and bodies need. With sleep come refreshment, energy and a will to live. Sound sleep allows us to reduce stress, to refocus and to regenerate our body organs. Lack of sleep has been associated with a shorter lifespan, moody behavior, poor immunity, chronic fatigue and affects every aspect of our health.

Lack of natural healing methods

As I am a strong advocate of natural medicine and drug-free healing methods, I strongly believe that conventional medicine with its rampant use of drugs including antibiotics, pain medications, anti-inflammatory drugs and others is not the way to go if you are interested in long-term health. We have seen the effects and we should learn from our mistakes. While modern medicine has its merits and often is life saving for acute or emergency situations, I do not feel that long-term drug therapy for chronic conditions such as back pain, high blood pressure, migraine headaches, stomach problems or others is a responsible solution for our growing health problems. Remember to search for the cause of health problems, not just the symptoms. With the new resurgence of natural healing methods like nutritional therapy, body therapies like Bowen therapy, herbals as well as many others, we now have so many natural alternatives to explore. Please read my book, *For Your Eyes Only* if you are interested in natural ways of diagnosing disease. Believe that the body can heal itself if given what it requires and give your body the best possible chance for recovery. Just as you would not want to ingest anything but natural foods, use natural healing methods that keep the body clean from drugs and contaminants and support the healing process in a natural way.

Lack of time in a natural environment and with animals

When was the last time that you spent time in a park, in the mountains or by the ocean?

This kind of therapy should be used by anyone who has any kind of chronic health problem as well as those who want to prevent health problems in the future. Energy from nature around us has powers of healing that we are only starting to understand. Spending time in the sun is very healthy if it is not in the peak hours between 10 a.m and 3 p.m. on summer days. We need the sun to produce Vitamin D and for our skin to breathe it needs to be exposed to the air. Synthetic clothing blocks our skin's ability to breathe and as it is an important detoxification organ it slows its ability to rid the body of toxins and harmful waste products. Several cases of acne and skin diseases like eczema have significantly improved when exposed to fresh air, sun and nature. If you suffer from health conditions including backaches, migraines, cancer or depression, get out to nature as soon as you can. Your mind and body will thank you for it. Spend time with animals as well as they are known to have phenomenal healing energy.

Lack of satisfying and challenging work

I believe that as human beings we all have a need for satisfying and challenging work.

Some of us require employment as doctors while others find satisfaction as mothers or housewives. It doesn't matter what you do just as long as you are happy doing it. I have found that many of my clients who do work for the wrong reasons or are unhappy with their working lives will have associated health problems.

Lack of balance and harmony

A balanced life is a combination of satisfying work, good friends, family and shared experiences. Equal time should be allotted for hobbies, for relaxation, for exercise and recreation, for family, friends and relationships. Any extremes that begin to show up indicate that our lives are not in balance and we are paving the way to signs of potential health problems. When all the forces including the physical, mental and spiritual are in balance with one another, a state of harmony is achieved. In this state we are best equipped to tackle problems that we encounter in life, to build friendships and relationships with others and to achieve optimum health.

Lack of positive thinking and motivation

Positive thinking is important for our physical and mental health. I believe that we should accept failures in our lives and learn from our mistakes and find the energy to look forward to the future. We cannot expect that our paths will always be paved with gold but we can try to look at the positive side of things no matter how difficult life can be. When we start thinking negatively our energy levels decrease, we lose motivation and reason to live. Our health is one of the first indicators of the effect of this decreased psychological energy. Our physical bodies are intertwined with our mental processes so positive thinking often determines how quickly we recover from injuries or disease.

Lack of learning, creativity, adventure and change

I believe that we all have a great capacity and requirement to learn. Most of us though reach a point in our lives where we begin to stagnate. It often shows up as boredom or dissatisfaction in our jobs. We tend to fall into a routine, learn it well but do not move forward. If you are feeling this way, take a chance and make a change. Explore your creativity. Start something completely brand new or take a course and learn what you have always wanted to learn. Exercise your mind with books and live through new experiences. Learning is an adventure and it can take you to places that you have always dreamed about. Do not allow fear to keep you in the safety zone where you know it all too well. Venture out! Life is about taking chances and living through experiences. This is how we learn, and how we move forward. A well-balanced healthy life involves change and learning.

Lack of acceptance and forgiveness

A healthy holistic lifestyle involves more than just the physical. Often I have seen in practice the effect of emotional blocks on the healing process. For some it is not possible to overcome serious disease unless those emotional barriers are broken down. I believe that life begins when you accept who you are and when you accept those who are around you. We are all different; we each have different roads to take. It's not an easy task but we have to respect our differences. I believe that true health and happiness only will come when we accept who we are and what role we play in this life.

The act of forgiveness is one of the greatest cleansers of our mind, body and spirit. When we forgive others, we accept that people are not perfect and make mistakes just as we do. When we forgive, we show a depth of acceptance and understanding. Only after forgiveness can there be release of negative feelings such as anger or resentment. These negative emotions often form blocks that affect our physical and psychological health.

Lack of the sense of spirituality and belief

The stressors of modern day life have left many searching for meaning, value, purpose and most of all, a deeper connection to self, others and the world around us. This is a time to explore our spiritual side. Spirituality can bring meaning into our lives. It has no doctrine or formal rules like religion, but is that part of us that longs for fulfillment. It can be prayer, meditation or contemplation of anything and everything that relates to the sense of being. Spirituality is a natural and essential part of all aspects of our everyday lives.

Holistic health involves the physical, mental as well as spiritual aspects of who we are.

Belief has always been a strong universal healer whether it is belief in God, in yourself, in others or in a worthy cause. When we stay true to our beliefs and convictions we stay in tune with our purpose in life. Belief often gives us a reason for living.

Lack of love, quality relationships and true happiness

The human need to love and to be loved is undoubtedly the most important holistic need of all. A lack of love in life is often associated with heart problems, stress, migraines, hormonal problems and many other physical manifestations. Without love we lose our will to live and lose our life path. A loss of a life partner or friend can often be devastating to our emotional and physical well-being. The emotion we call love is the essence of our existence and a requirement in our life in order to achieve true happiness.

As human beings we need contact with others. Relationships include the ties we have with our family members, our friends and loved ones. It includes those that are plutonic and those that are passionate or sexual. Relationships with others bring happiness, fulfillment and improved health. It is commonly and scientifically known that quality relationships add years to our lives.

Lack of hope or dreams

Where there is hope there is strong belief that a change for the better is possible. Hope gives us the opportunity to foresee a change before it actually happens. It gives us motivation, drive, a reason to live, an open path ahead of us and an opportunity to fulfill our dreams. When we lose hope, we lose our wings, we lose faith and the path in front of us becomes foggy. Our body, mind and spirit suffer.

If you are interested in learning about holistic healing needs and your powers of intuition, please read my *Holistic Healing Cards* and handbook.

BOWEN THERAPY

Tom Bowen's gift to the world

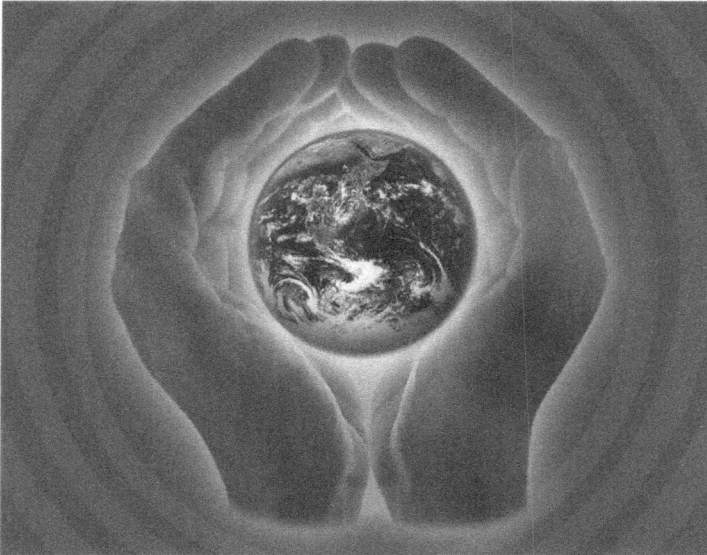

Part 2

How it began and how it works

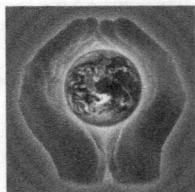

Who was Tom Bowen?
The History of his Method

Chapter

4

I never knew Tom Bowen. I really do wish I had had the honor to because to me he represented a humble man with a high moral sense of honesty, a genuine compassion for mankind, a passion for hard work and whose method clearly encompassed all the important principles of holistic healing that I believe in. Although his physical being has left us long ago, I believe that his spirit endures and remains close to those who have followed in his footsteps. His genuine compassion for human beings and his drive to help whoever he could through his care for the sick and disabled has been a great inspiration to me as well as the thousands across the globe who have chosen to carry on to teach or perform his pioneering work.

Those human elements are rare to find in today's world of modern medicine and drug therapy, where things just seem to get more and more complicated and many results are doubtful at best. In simplicity there is always beauty and the simplistic genius of Tom Bowen's unique method involved a series of moves on the body that has revolutionized the way many now view health care around the world. The miraculous work that has helped thousands and touched countless others the world over owes so much to this man's tireless efforts, who continued to refine his method right up to the last day of his death.

The principle of his method, known generally around the world today as Bowen therapy was to instigate a change in the body which would reactivate the body's innate healing capabilities and allow it to heal itself. Through his methods and his enormously successful practice, Tom Bowen was able to do this so well that he became famous during his lifetime in Australia and a legend after his death the whole world over.

Thomas Ambrose Bowen was born in April 1916 in Brunswick, Australia and died in October 1982. He devoted a lifetime to pioneering and developing a unique and innovative healing approach in Geelong, Australia that he referred to as soft tissue therapy. Although he had no formal medical training, in 1975 it was documented by the Australian Government in a survey on natural therapies that he was treating around 13,000 patients per year, a remarkable number considering that the majority would only receive two treatments each.

Tom left school at the age of 14 and worked at a series of laboring jobs eventually taking up his father's trade of carpentry and working as a general hand at Geelong cement works. It was at that time that he began to treat people, eventually expanding to a full time practice.

He started practicing massage for local junior football clubs and treated the general public after hours until his practice began to flourish. Soon his practice grew to amazing proportions and it is said that he treated between 50 to 60 patients a day. He regularly treated disabled people free of charge and would make home visits to those who could not reach his clinic.

Tom Bowen did not believe in long-term treatments and the majority received only two or three treatments each. He soon became famous for curing the incurable and his reputation grew in leaps and bounds. He worked on refining his techniques over many years and it is said that he continued to develop his method even up to the last day before his death.

It has been often said of Tom Bowen that he had about six long-term students who learned and studied from him. One of them was Oswald Rensch, who after Bowen's death was responsible for first teaching his interpretation of Bowen's method and spreading the word to many countries of the world. I had the opportunity to briefly meet Ossie Rensch when I lived in Australia during the time when I first began practicing the Bowen method and found his passion for the Bowen technique very inspirational. It was Tom Bowen's healing method that finally inspired me to bring his technique to the

Czech republic where I became the first to gain its accreditation by the Ministry of Education in 1999 and soon began teaching my interpretation.

Despite the popularity of Bowen therapy, very little is known of Tom Bowen himself or of how he developed his method, which has further added to the mystery behind this method. It has been often said that he was a relatively quiet man who had a sincere concern for humanity as well as a passion for sports especially swimming and he was actively involved in coaching young people. He married in the early nineteen forties and had three children. His health was not very good, was a diabetic who lost his leg and wore hearing aids, being almost deaf in both ears. He eventually lost his other leg just weeks before his death. He considered himself an osteopath but was unregistered as he had no formal training and after being invited to test for registration as an osteopath, he failed. Despite his miraculous method that had treated thousands, he was refused membership to the osteopathic council in 1982, a major disappointment to him as it meant that his patients could not claim his services on their medical insurance.

Many accounts have reported that Tom Bowen had what was described as a hypersensitivity of the fingers and hands which allowed him to find blockages in the muscular and nervous systems of the body. He claimed that he could sense nerve vibrations and would often feel burning sensations on his fingers that were so hot that he would have to leave the room and cool them down under cold running water. His work did not stop with just humans as he also achieved great success for his methods on animals such as racehorses.

Tom Bowen was also said to have an amazing ability to diagnose at an instant. He could tell just by looking at an individual what was wrong and the cause of their problem. It has been said that he looked at how the patient's jaw was set to determine his diagnosis.

Today, over 20 years after his death, the legend of Tom Bowen is still alive and grows year by year with each success story. The method that started in Australia has now reached well over 25 countries around the world. Due to its amazing success the Bowen method continues to grow in popularity among a variety of therapist groups including osteopaths, chiropractors, physiotherapists, massage therapists, doctors, dentists, kinesiologists, sports doctors, psychologists, naturopaths and many other health professionals.

I sincerely believe that as long as those who have carried on his work perform it with genuine compassion and with honest intentions, as did Tom Bowen, the method will continue to perform the same miracles for which Tom was famous for back in Australia. Perhaps we will never really unveil the mystery of how and why his method works so well for so many people. Perhaps it is not so important to know but to just be grateful for Tom Bowen's pioneering efforts.

I would personally like to thank you Tom Bowen, on behalf of my students and patients for your gift that you have shared and passed on to me so that I can continue to teach, to write about and to carry on the work that you started.

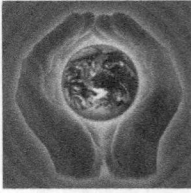

What is Bowen Therapy?

Now that you have gained some insight into some of the reasons why pain and disease occur as well as who Tom Bowen was, let's take a closer look at the meaning of Bowen therapy.

This fascinating method is a dynamic bodywork technique that often results in rapid and lasting relief from pain and discomfort. As I have previously mentioned, it is safe to use on anyone, from newborns to the elderly and provides benefits from conditions such as sports injuries to a variety of chronic health problems.

I think the best way to describe Bowen therapy is first to say what it is and then what it is not.

Bowen therapy is:

- a very gentle method and can often be very relaxing

- a method that empowers the body's own healing resources

- a holistic method that works on the entire body

- safe and effective for newborns to the elderly

- a series of gentle pressure point moves that are manually applied over specific muscles, tendons, nerves and ligaments with specific designated resting periods

- a technique that uses soft-tissue manipulation to stimulate specific reflex points in the body

- an effective method that relaxes muscle tension without aggressive manipulation

- a method that stimulates the blood circulation and lymphatic flow without the pushing of fluids as in typical lymphatic drainage or sports massage

- a method that addresses misalignments in the body without aggressive manipulation of bones and joints as in chiropractic medicine.

- a relaxation method that stimulates the nervous system, reduces anxiety and nervous tension and commonly results in feelings of increased energy and vitality

- a natural method that uses no needles, electricity, heating or vibration pads

- a method that often evokes psychological release

- a method that can be applied over clothes or directly on the skin

Bowen therapy is <u>not</u>:

- classical massage, acupressure, chiropractic, energy work or lymphatic massage although it comprises aspects of each of these disciplines making it a complete new method of its own

- a method that employs deep pressure or rapid or sharp aggressive moves

- a method that uses oils or lubricants on the skin

- a method that employs the uses of needles, electricity, heating or vibration or any other adjunct equipment

Interpretations of Tom Bowen's work

What method is the real true Bowen?

Today there are literally hundreds of interpretations of Tom Bowen's method around the world, some which use Bowen in their name and others that have been given new names. Some methods claim to be true representations of Bowen's method and others have incorporated new methods or combined methods from other disciplines. Whatever the case, each interpretation of Bowen's method will always differ in some ways to the original because the only true version of Bowen is the method that Tom Bowen knew himself which no one can justifiably replicate. As time passes his method will evolve probably just as his method would have evolved if he were still alive and working on it today. I believe that Tom Bowen left us with some pioneering work that he had started but had not completed and he left the rest for us to find it out. I also believe that just as it is important to remember the basic techniques that Tom Bowen has taught us, it is also important to experiment and expand on his work as well. We can equate it in some way by the fact that we all start by learning the same words of a language, including sentence structure and grammar but we all go on to write different books.

This book on Bowen therapy is of course my book and in some ways my interpretation of Tom Bowen's method that was taught to me by some of the early pioneers of this method in Australia. Although it seeks to come as close as possible to the original techniques of Tom Bowen, there have naturally evolved slight differences in combinations of sequences that have been developed as a result of my many years of clinical practice. In my opinion, I believe that they serve to be only slight improvements to the original method.

Bowen therapy has worked for me in a high percentage of cases; in many instances it has performed what even doctors have called miracles. It has often prevented the need for surgery as well as the need for unnecessary drugs and medications. I have witnessed dramatic improvements in digestion and other internal body processes with its use as well as improved mental well-being. It forms an integral component of holistic health, that of touch that is often deficient in modern society and has the ability to deal with imbalances in the body that are commonly the cause of many health problems. As almost everyone subjects themselves to some form of abuse on the body, whether physical or mental, I firmly believe that Bowen therapy can be a very positive health experience for almost everyone.

What is Bowen therapy? Just ask the thousands of patients that have achieved relief from their pain and other chronic problems around the world, whose incredible results have baffled even the greatest medical minds of today. It is that wonderful gift that Tom Bowen has left us, a method, which resets the body and builds a firm foundation so that it can begin healing itself.

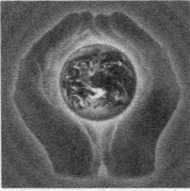

Theories of how Bowen Therapy may work

As the Bowen method spreads rapidly across the globe, many questions have arisen as to why certain moves are used and the rationale of how they work. Unfortunately most of these questions have still been left unanswered. If Tom Bowen was alive today I am sure a large percentage of the Bowen community would love to know how he developed his technique and what it actually does in the body. Unfortunately we are only left now with speculation and theories of how the Bowen method may work.

Perhaps we are really not meant to understand everything that we see but to be just satisfied with that it works. I can't help to think of all the alternative methods of healing that have been scorned and dismissed by modern medicine just because they could never be proved by scientific tests. All the laws that have banned natural healing methods over the years just so that we could achieve this low grade medical care that we are forced to accept today. We will all pay for our lack of being open to new ideas and our lack of abiding by the laws of nature. For all those closed minds out there, remember one thing, we have only scraped the surface of having an understanding about how our bodies work and function and what affects their ability. Modern medicine unfortunately is in its infancy and despite its claims of medical advances, its rampant use of chemical drugs to treat disease can be only seen as primitive and damaging to our long-term health. This, I hope you can see is not holistic medicine. If it were so successful we would not be suffering from alarmingly increasing rates of cancer, diabetes, asthma, migraine headaches and allergies among a host of other chronic problems.

As we venture into areas that we cannot fully explain, we cannot help but to feel a sense of mystery with what Tom Bowen has left us. The Bowen method is as mysterious as its founder and I believe holds many secrets for our long-term health and well-being. Let's take a look at some possible theories that have been suggested for how the Bowen method may work.

Nerve stimulation theory

The Bowen move that is administrated to the body triggers an impulse in the nervous system that activates a host of communication channels to and from the brain which results in nerve reflexes that relax and balance body muscles, relieve muscle spasms and stimulate the function of body organs. The result is increased circulation of blood, lymph and energy flow in the body. Bowen therapy helps the body remember how to heal through its stimulation of its sense organs, the proprioceptors that are used for fine movement and balance. The messages sent to the nervous system return from the brain where they act to remind the body to regain normal movement in our joints, muscles, and tendons.

Vibrational theory

The unique rolling action of the Bowen method over specific locations on the body generates vibrational patterns at specific frequencies. These frequencies correspond to specific areas of the body depending on where the moves are made. Just as the tuning of a piano or guitar strings, the Bowen method assists in rebalancing and tuning the body's system. In generating ideal vibrational patterns the body can reach a state of homeostasis or harmony. In this way it provides a catalyst for the healing process.

Meridian theory

The locations of each of the Bowen moves correlate with research into the meridian energy system, acupressure and acupuncture points. Several of the moves are located along acupuncture meridians or on specific points used in acupuncture, which are known to stimulate and balance the body's energy levels. As we know with acupuncture there exist meridians in the body which may explain why a Bowen move on a distant site on the body will trigger a reflex, or reaction in a location elsewhere.

Stress release theory

The body endures tremendous stress during times of physical trauma, poor posture and deep emotional conflicts. This affects the autonomic nervous system and is responsible for stress reactions such as the "fight or flight" reaction, which reduces the ability of the body to rest, recover and regenerate. The Bowen method balances the autonomic nervous system so that the stress dominated sympathetic side is reduced. As a result or this stress release, muscle tension decreases, hypersensitivity of the nerves is reduced, acute pain is relieved and healing is accelerated.

It seems that it is human nature to try to understand all that we can and to attempt to prove any new technique by scientific methods. Remember, there are just so many factors that influence our health and they go far beyond just the physical. If we accept the fact that we currently know just a fraction of how the body works, we will maintain an open mind to new ideas and learning will come as we gain more experience. A closed mind learns nothing.

Whatever the reason why Bowen performs as it does, we know that other forces are at work than just what we can physically see. Whether the Bowen method stimulates nervous impulses, alters vibrational patterns in the body, activates the meridian energy system, or releases the stress reaction, we know it works in mysterious ways that we are only just starting to understand. Just because we cannot prove a theory does not mean we should stop performing the Bowen method. As it has helped so many thousands of people around the world to deal with chronic pain and ill health and has no known negative side effects, I believe despite our inability to find an explanation of how it works, it still deserves a firm place in our current health system.

BOWEN THERAPY

Tom Bowen's gift to the world

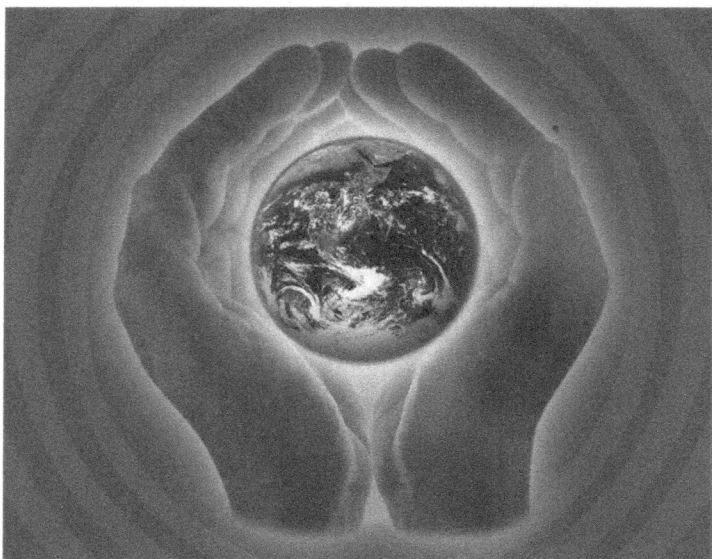

Part 3

Useful information to know <u>before</u> your session

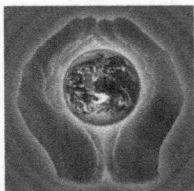

Nutrition, Health and Bowen Therapy

Chapter 7

In my opinion, nutrition works hand in hand with the Bowen method and together they produce the greatest long-lasting results. Although this book does not cover nutrition in any kind of detail, I would recommend reading my book, *The Eye for an Eye Diet* if you are interested in a comprehensive holistic view on all aspects of nutrition.

Nutrition is essential to our existence, without it we cannot achieve optimal health. We also cannot expect that our bodies will regenerate or that our old cells will be replaced with new ones if our diet is not well balanced. This means that your sore back, migraine headache or knee problem will not be cured by the Bowen method alone. Bowen therapy will activate the energy and circulatory channels in the body and clear the way so that the body can start to heal itself but if given only poor nutrition, the results will not last very long.

Therefore, I would always recommend taking a close look at what you eat and ensure adequate water intake especially if you have any kind of chronic health problems such as chronic back pain, digestive difficulties, hormonal problems, arthritic complaints, breathing problems, poor skin health or heart conditions.

Take a look at what I call the **seven essential processes of life**. The first and probably most important essential process is INGESTION and it depends on what we take into the body in the form of nutrition, sunlight, the air and various kinds of energy around us. We also require effective DIGESTION so that the food we eat can be broken down to smaller units to allow for ABSORPTION of nutrients into the blood. Adequate CIRCULATION is essential to transport these absorbed nutrients to their final destination, the cells. There, through the process of UTILIZATION, they can provide en-

48

ergy for cellular processes. Cells also produce waste products that need to be removed through DETOXIFICATION organs like our digestive system, liver, kidneys, lungs, lymphatic system and skin. Only when all these essential life processes are working well and receiving the nutrition they need, can the body activate its process of REGENERATION, which allows old worn out cells to be replaced by healthy new ones. So you see, what you eat or what you ingest is critical to your body's ability to heal and regenerate.

This means that you cannot properly heal your aching back without the regeneration of muscles, tendons, bone and ligaments. You cannot properly heal your migraine headache without adequate circulation and detoxification. You cannot properly heal your arthritic complaints or any chronic health problem without the smooth functioning of each of these essential processes of life. Avoid looking for a quick fix to your health problems. Your body needs to create a healing environment in order to regenerate. An effective healing environment is far better achieved by Bowen therapy, which activates the body's healing processes in combination with good nutrition and exercise that supports each of the essential life processes.

What constitutes a well-balanced diet that will promote regeneration?

Take the time to time to read through this important nutritional advice.

1. Ensure that the food you eat is free of chemicals, colors and other preservatives to decrease the burden on the body's detoxification process.

2. Make sure to reduce simple and low fiber complex carbohydrates, especially sugar and consume more high-fiber complex carbohydrates that contain fiber preferably in their unprocessed, natural raw form.

3. Ensure quality protein in your diet that includes all the amino acids but not in excessive amounts as found in most

Western high meat-eating cultures. Try to achieve protein intake from healthier sources such as fish, nuts and plant sources.

4. Remember that fats are essential in our diet but in order to
    lower cholesterol and stay lean and healthy, they should not
    be excessive. Polyunsaturated and mono-unsaturated are best
    and the intake of saturated fats (meat and milk products) and
    trans fatty acids (French fries, chips and cookies) in the diet
    should be reduced.

5. Water is one of the most important nutrients that we ingest.
    We cannot live very long without water and the majority of
    our body is composed of it. Low water intake is associated
    with many health problems and we need to drink more water
    especially if we consume coffee, black tea or alcohol. Find
    natural sources of water and use filters for tap water to reduce
    contaminants such as chlorine. Drink a minimum of one un-
    sweetened, un-carbonated glass per day for every 9 kilograms
    / 20 pounds of body weight. As the Bowen method often re-
    sults in the release of built-up toxins, it is critical that you
    increase water intake to allow these toxins to flush out of the
    body.

6. Increase your intake of fiber by eating more whole grains,
    fruits and vegetables. Fiber increases the bulk of the food con-
    tents and increases bowel transit time as well as removing
    cholesterol and fats from the body and slowing down the ab-
    sorption of sugars. Many health problems are associated with
    lack of fiber in the diet including constipation, cancer of the
    colon, hemorrhoids and high blood cholesterol.

7. Ensure a well-balanced nutritional diet that supplies adequate
    protein, carbohydrates, fats, vitamins, minerals and fiber. En-
    sure that your diet consists of mainly vegetables, whole grains,
    fruits and berries, some fish, poultry, eggs, nuts and legumes,
    and minimal milk products, sweets, white flour, potatoes, al-
    cohol and red meat. Include oils such as olive oil but use
    butter sparingly.

8. Minimize the amount of processed or altered food in your diet and prepare food by reducing cooking time and temperature so that it contains the highest amount of nutritional value. Avoid cooking methods such as frying, grilling or microwaving. Eat at least 60 percent of your dietary fruits and vegetables in the raw form.

9. Avoid ingesting contaminants along with food, which impose additional burdens on the body's detoxification system and slow down the process of regeneration. Try to purchase organic produce and free-range eggs and poultry, adequately wash fruits and vegetables, limit canned and processed foods and source clean drinking water.

10. Avoid excess milk products, margarine, smoked, salty or pickled foods, refined white flour or sugar products, instant and fast foods and excess animal protein. Food items like artificial sweeteners and soft drinks and many condiments have very little or no nutritional value in your diet. Ingestion of many of these foods has been associated with several health problems and I would recommend using them minimally in your diet.

11. Avoid excess alcohol, caffeine, salt, saturated fat and white sugar. These foods cause imbalances in the body chemistry and cause cravings. Try to avoid or limit these foods in your diet and opt for natural foods that will balance your body's nutritional needs.

12. Increase the intake of healing foods that include dark green vegetables and sprouts, fresh fruits and berries, avocado, eggs, figs and dates, nuts and seeds, garlic, fish, olive oil, fresh vegetable juices, grapes and chlorella.

Remember, if you are considering Bowen therapy to help assist with your health problems or chronic back pain, ensure healthy nutrition to allow the body the greatest chance to heal itself through natural means.

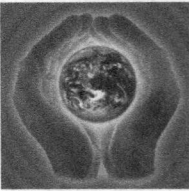

When should you consider undergoing Bowen Therapy?

The decision to undergo Bowen therapy depends on your current state of health, the type of health problem you have or how important preventative health is to you. Virtually all types of conditions can be assisted with the Bowen Method.

Here is a list of health conditions for which the Bowen method has been used very effectively.

Allergies

Ankle sprains

Anxiety

Arthritis

Asthma

Back and neck pain

Back pain during pregnancy

Bedwetting in children

Breast tenderness

Breathing difficulties

Bronchitis

Cancer

Chest pain

Circulatory problems

Cold fingers and feet

Colds and flu

Colicky infants

Constipation

Cramps

Cystitis

Cysts

Depression

Diarrhea

Digestive problems

Dizziness and nausea

Ear infections

Edema

Eyesight

Facial nerve paralysis

Fatigue

Fever

Frozen shoulder

Groin

Gynecological problems

Hay fever

Headaches

Hearing

Heart problems

Hernia

High and low blood pressure

Hormonal problems

Incontinence

Indigestion

Infertility

Insomnia

Jaw imbalances

Joint problems

Kidney problems

Knee problems

Liver weakness

Low immunity

Lymphatic congestion

Mastitis

Menopause symptoms

Menstrual pain

Migraines

Nerve pain

Nerve problems

Obesity

Osteoporosis

Premenstrual pain

Problems with lactation

Prostate gland problems

Scoliosis and curvatures of the spine

Sinus congestion

Skin problems

Sleep disorders

Stress

Swollen ankles

Tennis elbow

Tingling feelings in the arms or legs

Tinnitus

Toothaches

Upper respiratory infections

Urinary tract infections

Varicose veins

Wrist problems

If you have any of the above health problems, the Bowen method may provide assistance. Your Bowen therapist will advise you what sequences are best for your condition, those that will stimulate your body's healing processes and that can provide lasting relief from your health conditions.

Times when you should consider undergoing Bowen Therapy

- When you have any of the above health conditions

- When you find that you are getting sick more and more often

- When you are tired and run down

- When you are suffering from stress or anxiety

- When you suffer from bouts of depression

- When you feel any kind of pain

- When you are having difficulties losing or gaining weight

- When you need a boost in your energy levels

- When you have suffered any kind of intense emotional distress

Common questions:

Do you have to be a certain age to undergo Bowen therapy?

No, the Bowen method is safe for everyone. It can be applied even to infants and the elderly as well as those with chronic health problems such as cancer or diabetes.

Many types of massage are not recommended for the elderly as they tend to have brittle bones and weak musculature which can in some cases create problems and injury. The Bowen method is so gentle that the chance of injury is virtually impossible.

Does it make sense to undergo Bowen therapy when I currently do not have any health problems?

The answer lies in the importance of prevention. Just because you currently do not have any pain or discomfort does not mean that you will not have it in the future. The Bowen method is as effective in assisting in the prevention of disease as it is with dealing with disease. Regular Bowen sessions can strengthen your immune system as the lymphatic system will stay clear, your circulation will be stimulated so that your organs receive the blood supply they need and the nervous system will be activated allowing the functioning of all body systems. All in all, the Bowen method along with good nutrition and regular exercise is an excellent way to prevent disease.

What about if I am pregnant?

Although there are some minimal contraindications for using the Bowen method during pregnancy, as you will see when we discuss the coccyx procedure, most sequences can be used safely and are beneficial during pregnancy. Some sequences can even be applied while you are on your side. Ask your Bowen therapist for details if you are pregnant.

What if I have acute back pain? Can I still undergo Bowen therapy?

Yes, often the Bowen method can provide quick relief for acute back and neck pain and allow a healing environment for faster recovery.

Can I undergo the Bowen method if I have a fever?

Yes, the Bowen method can assist in reducing fever, in relieving aches and pains and in helping the clearing of the lymphatic system to strengthen the immune system. In this way the duration of your flu or disease can be significantly reduced.

How many Bowen sessions are required?

Usually the minimum amount of recommended sessions is three but you may require up to ten or more in certain chronic cases. After that it is a good idea to allow your body some time to heal itself. Bowen sessions can be repeated again throughout the year for maintenance, lymphatic drainage and in times of stress or fatigue. Your therapist will advise you of the best way that Bowen therapy can assist you with your health problem.

I hope that after you read through this book, you will be convinced, as I am, that Bowen therapy is one of the greatest discoveries in health care today. Its most noted benefits lie in its universal application to almost all health conditions and its safe use for all ages, making it a truly wonderful holistic method of its own.

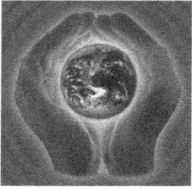

The benefits and positive effects of Bowen Therapy

We have already mentioned a few of the many benefits of the Bowen method including the numerous health conditions it can assist and its universal application. Here is a complete list of benefits and the positive effects that can be realized after your Bowen session. It should be noted that every one of us is different and therefore the effects of Bowen therapy can also vary among clients.

Pain Relief

Probably the greatest reason why most clients will undergo the Bowen method is for relief of pain. Pain can occur for many reasons including injury, infection or inflammation, degeneration of body organs and bones, or poor circulation and nerve innervation. Pain is an indication of imbalance in the body and a warning sign that the body requires assistance. The Bowen method often significantly reduces pain often after only the first session.

Lymphatic drainage

Bowen therapy has an indirect effect of stimulating the lymphatic system. As the lymphatic system is prone to become congested reducing the effectiveness of the immune system, lymphatic drainage is beneficial. Bowen therapy with its combination of effective sequences provides sufficient lymphatic drainage.

Works holistically and allows the body to heal itself

The Bowen method does not just focus on a specific health problem but also works on the entire body at the same time. Circulation throughout all the organ systems is stimulated ensuring improvements in the body's ability to self-heal.

Safe for children and the elderly

Even young children can benefit from the therapeutic effects of the Bowen method. The elderly can be assured that this method is safe and virtually painless for even the most sensitive individuals. Where other rigorous methods of treatment are contraindicated, the gentle effective action of the Bowen method can be used for all types of people.

Moves can be applied even over clothing

There is no need to fully undress when undergoing Bowen treatment. One of the greatest advantages is that the Bowen moves can be applied even over light clothing. However for comfort, it is recommended to remove heavy clothing and to wear loose clothing like sweat pants rather than jeans or tight pants.

Stimulates energy flow and circulation

The flow of energy throughout the body is something that is very difficult to ascertain. Bowen clients often report feelings of warmth in areas of the body, which indicate that circulation is stimulated and that energy flow in the body is attempting to balance itself. Often poor circulation is the cause of a variety of health problems. Once energy flow and circulation is restored to weak areas of the body, a positive healing environment is established, once again activating the natural healing processes.

Balances muscles tension

Unbalanced muscle tension is often the cause of pain, poor flexibility or poor posture. The Bowen method is very effective, through its use of positive and negative moves, to reduce muscle tension in areas of the body, often reducing pain, inflammation and swelling.

Reduces stress

Stress is one of the greatest silent killers of our civilization. It is responsible for contributing to so many health problems including heart disease, high blood pressure and migraine headaches, just to name a few. One of the miraculous benefits of the Bowen method is that by reducing muscle tension and improving the flow of energy in the body, the client can much better handle stress so that it does not damage the body. Clients often report feelings of rejuvenation, increased energy and lightness.

Can be used for chronic health problems or sports injuries

The Bowen method is advantageous for a variety of chronic problems, even those including internal conditions such as constipation, kidney weakness or digestive difficulties. Those who have been injured in sporting activities such as knee injuries, ankle sprains, shoulder or groin injuries can benefit greatly from the Bowen method. In some cases even surgical operations can be avoided.

Improves digestion and absorption of nutrients

Bowen clients often report improvements from constipation or stomach problems. By improving circulation and reducing muscle tension in the body, the digestive system will be better prepared to absorb nutrients that will reach the cells for faster healing. A combination of Bowen therapy with improvements in diet and lifestyle can work miracles.

Improves breathing ability and absorption of oxygen in the lungs

Often those who suffer from asthma, bronchitis, emphysema or other respiratory disorders find relief with the Bowen method. Improved circulation and reduction of muscle tension will increase pulmonary capacity assisting the lungs in gas exchange.

Rids the body of harmful toxins

The Bowen method achieves detoxification of harmful toxins by stimulating the lymphatic system, improving circulation and activating the kidneys to do their job better. Harmful toxins that stay in the body can often lead to chronic fatigue, inflammation, headaches and other degenerative diseases.

Often improves psychological problems

Bowen clients often report improvement in a variety of psychological conditions such as depression, anxiety and stress. Many find that they feel calmer and find it easier to cope with emotional trauma. The Bowen method can assist in some cases to allow deeply suppressed emotions the chance to surface.

Improves skin function

By activating the body's detoxification channels, which also include the skin, Bowen therapy often results in better skin health. Improvements in eczema, acne, and other skin irritations are commonly seen after a period of time once the skin begins to regain its function to clear toxins from the body as well as its ability to breathe.

Can assist in the removal of cysts

Cysts in some cases have been found to disappear after Bowen sessions. This is not a surprise as once detoxification is improved and lymphatic drainage is achieved, the body regains its ability to clear wastes.

Improves the posture of the body

Poor posture is often the cause of pain, deformities in the spine and even psychological problems. The Bowen method releases muscle tension in the body so that homeostasis is regained and poor posture is often corrected. It is important though to maintain regular exercise and to not strain the spine with unnatural movements and positions.

Improves the healing capability of tissue

Finally, improving detoxification and circulation and stimulating energy flow radically improve the healing capability of tissues. This means that injuries will heal faster and degenerated muscles, ligaments and organs, will find it easier to regenerate.

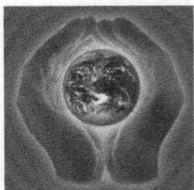

Important information to tell your Bowen therapist

A common error that we tend to make when we visit the doctor or therapist is to withhold information about our health status. What we forget to understand is that the more they know about what problems plague us, the greater assistance they can provide. Do not conceal information and try to share as much information about your health as you can. Even symptoms that you may feel are minor are important as they can uncover hidden clues to what may be causing your aches and pains or other health problems. Here are some questions that your Bowen therapist will most likely ask you before you begin your sessions. Be prepared to offer this information even if they do not ask.

Is this the first time you have had this problem or is it a chronic problem that you have had for an extended period of time?

Generally the more chronic the problem the more there are other associated problems that exist. Your Bowen therapist will try to identify the causes of your health problem and plan the best combination of sequences, using specific procedures from the Bowen method.

Are you undergoing any other therapy for this problem?

It is usually advisable when undergoing the Bowen method, to not engage in any other manipulative therapy including physiotherapy, chiropractic, massage, acupuncture or acupressure. Your Bowen therapist will probably ask you this question before you begin your sessions. It is important to reduce the amount of signals that are sent to the body so that the Bowen method can do its work effectively. It will also allow the Bowen therapist to be able to ascertain if a procedure is working or if other procedures should be used. It is advisable to refrain from any body therapy for five days before your first Bowen session to five days after your last Bowen session.

Are you taking any medications?

Having knowledge of whether any medications are currently being taken will give the Bowen therapist a background on your medical history.

What is your main complaint? What other complaints do you have?

Generally most of you will make an appointment for a Bowen session for a specific complaint, such as back pain. Take note of other signs of discomfort that you may have such as digestive difficulties, constipation, headaches or fatigue and share this information with your Bowen therapist.

What type of pain is it? Where does it originate? Is it an acute stabbing pain or a dull pain? How long have you had this pain?

It is important for the Bowen therapist to know what type of pain you are experiencing so that he or she can better ascertain the cause. The location of the pain as well as the intensity can provide valuable information.

Is this problem the result of an accident or injury?

Information on the cause of your health problem is useful for the Bowen therapist. If your complaint has been the result of accident of injury, make sure you let your Bowen therapist know.

Have you had any accidents or injuries in the past?

Past accidents or injuries often uncover hidden clues to health problems. Any imbalance that we have imposed on our bodies can create muscle tension often resulting in pain and inflammation.

Have you undergone any operations?

You may have undergone an operation many years ago that you may think is not related to your current problem or it may be an operation that has reduced the flexibility of the back, knee, shoulder or other area of the body. Whatever the situation, inform your Bowen therapist of all the operations you have had in the past. Again this information will allow him or her to choose the best combination of procedures to assist your problem.

Are you under any stress at the moment?

When confronted with this question, most of us are usually under at least some kind of stress in our lives, which is normal. If you are suffering from intense stress, emotional distress, depression or other psychological dysfunctions, inform your Bowen therapist.

Are you pregnant?

It is important to let your Bowen therapist know if you are pregnant as there are some procedures that should not be performed during pregnancy.

Are you drinking enough water? How much are you drinking daily?

Be honest about the amount of water you are drinking daily. It is very important at least during your Bowen sessions to increase your fluid intake as a large load of toxins are usually released through this method and need water to flush them out.

Do you have a well-balanced diet?

Often the root of many problems is the type of food we eat. By analyzing your diet, you may find what you are lacking which may be contributing to your current health problem.

Do you have any deformities, curvatures of the spine, scars?

Your Bowen therapist will often check the curvature of your back, your posture and other visible deformities. Let him or her know of any that you are aware of including scars from accidents or operations.

Do you have any skin problems?

Do not be embarrassed to reveal that you have any kind of skin disease. As Bowen therapy is often performed over light clothing, any skin problem may not be immediately evident. Let your Bowen therapist know of any skin infections, sensitivity or skin disease. This information will assist him or her to determine what procedures are necessary.

Do you have decreased flexibility during any types of movements?

Your Bowen therapist may take you through a few exercises to test your flexibility. If you are aware of any loss of range of movement around any of your joints, inform your Bowen therapist.

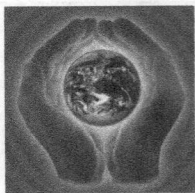

Essential information for Bowen clients, and contraindications

Here are 20 important points to know before your first Bowen session:

1. The Bowen method is a gentle, non-aggressive method and is safe to use for almost any health problem.

2. It is critical to drink a minimum of 1.5 liters of water daily especially between your Bowen therapy sessions. This will allow your detoxification organs to flush out wastes and toxins that are released by administration of the Bowen method.

3. The Bowen method does not treat any specific health problem but can assist the body to heal itself holistically.

4. No other type of body therapy including different types of massage, chiropractic, acupuncture, acupressure or physiotherapy, should be undertaken less than five days before your first Bowen session and five days after your last Bowen session. This is to allow Bowen to do its work without any interference or mixing of signals from other therapies.

5. Try not to talk too much during your Bowen session and allow your mind to relax and free yourself from any concerns or worries. This will allow for muscle tension release and activation of the body's healing processes.

6. Do not expect miracles overnight but allow Bowen to do its work in the body. Positive success depends a lot on what you do after your session.

7. Remember less is more. Too many procedures on the first day can promote more negative reactions especially if you

have chronic problems that have lasted for years. Do not try to convince your Bowen therapist to do more work on you than is necessary.

8. Your Bowen therapist will frequently stop the procedure to allow for 2-minute breaks or longer ones in some cases. They may also leave the room in some cases to allow the energy to work on your body. Do not be surprised, as this is part of the procedure of Bowen therapy.

9. If you feel any significant pain during your procedure, make sure to inform your Bowen therapist.

10. You may feel warmth in some areas during the Bowen session and some moves may feel over-sensitive. Be aware of this and inform your Bowen therapist when you encounter feelings like this.

11. The earliest that you can come for a second Bowen session is 5 days. Usually a week between sessions is ideal but should not exceed 10 days.

12. Do not bring your mobile or cellular phone in with you to your Bowen session. Avoid distracting interruptions so that you can concentrate on relaxing your mind and body.

13. A maximum of two people, you and your Bowen therapist, should be in the same room during the procedure. Other family members or friends should wait in the waiting room. The reason for this is again to ensure total relaxation and to not allow other energies from other people to interfere will the healing and muscle release process.

14. If you feel unwell, dizzy or nauseous during your Bowen session, please inform your therapist immediately.

15. The location of the moves for Bowen therapy are across most areas of the body, especially the lower and upper back, neck, legs, arms and head. You may be asked to turn over during your Bowen session or to turn your head from one side to the other.

16. The maximum number of times that one specific procedure should be performed on the body is twice during the same session.

17. The Bowen method works best when your muscles are in a fully relaxed state. This means that while lying on the table you should not be experiencing any pain or be in a position of discomfort as this causes your muscles to contract. Advise your Bowen therapist if you are not feeling relaxed and he or she will place you in a more comfortable position.

18. The average time for a Bowen massage is between 20 minutes and 40 minutes in most cases, depending on how many procedures are used and whether it is the first or following Bowen session.

19. You do not need to undress during a Bowen massage. It is advisable that you wear light clothing and loose pants to ensure greatest comfort and best results.

20. Most of the Bowen procedures are done while you are lying on your stomach or on your back. A few are performed while in a sitting or standing position.

Contraindications:

There are very few contraindications for the Bowen method but these two should be noted.

1. The **"coccyx procedure"** should not be performed on women who are pregnant.

2. The **"breast tenderness procedure"** should not be performed on women with silicone breast implants.

BOWEN THERAPY

Tom Bowen's gift to the world

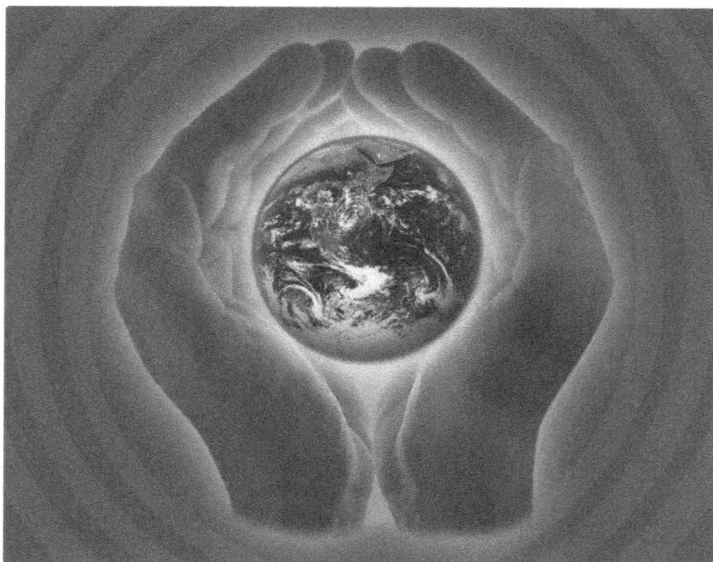

Part 4

The method, moves and sequences

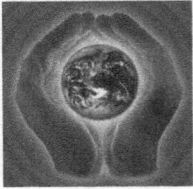

The Bowen move

Probably the most fundamental component of Bowen therapy is the move itself.

Although there are a variety of different types of moves and variations of moves used throughout the Bowen procedures on different parts of the body, the Bowen move in its basic form, differentiates the Bowen method from any other body therapy in the world.

Although the move appears simple, it usually takes quite a lot of training before it is effective and perfected. It is the essence of this move that utilizes a combination of positive and negative movements that stimulate the muscles, tendons and nerves. The very core of this basic move is what all the Bowen moves and procedures are based on.

In order for you to understand the Bowen move you need to become familiar with its 3 distinct parts. In essence, the first two parts are preparations for the last part, the move that is administered.

Part 1

Taking back the Skin Slack in the direction opposite to the move that is intended

Often this is difficult to learn at the start, as there is a common tendency to move not just the skin but the underlying structures as well. Therefore, it is very important to maintain a firm but light touch as you draw the skin slack back. In preparation for the move itself, the skin slack is drawn back in the opposite or negative direction to the move using the thumbs or fingers. Again the distance the skin can be pulled back depends on the individual. In some cases, you may feel the slack of the skin very easily and it will pull back a great deal, in others the skin may be very taught and when you pull back it may move only very little. It is important to not pull back any more than the skin allows and to avoid any kind of sliding of the fingers over the skin. Remember only very light pressure is needed to draw the skin slack back.

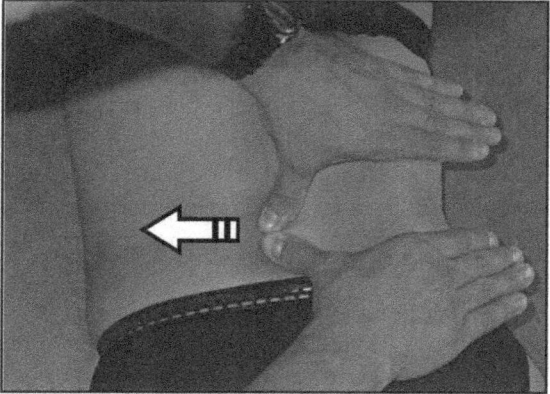

Part 2

Light pressure in the direction of the intended move

Once the skin slack is moved back, firm but light pressure is applied for a few seconds in the direction of the intended move.

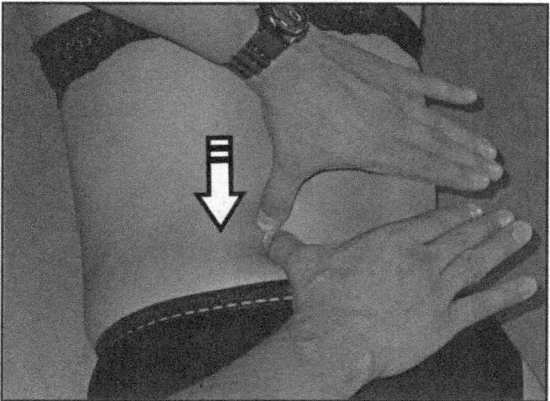

This allows the body to become prepared for the move itself and also allows the Bowen therapist to fully concentrate his or her efforts on administering the move accurately.

Part 3

The move itself, which consists of a rolling motion over the nerve, muscle, tendon or ligament

After the few seconds of light pressure, the Bowen therapist is ready to administer the Bowen move. In most cases, either both thumbs of each hand or both index fingers are used with the occasional heel of the hand or elbow, depending on the nature of the procedure. The important aspect to remember when performing the Bowen move is that even pressure is maintained throughout the whole movement. The Bowen move enables the transfer of information to the relevant area of the body, stimulating nerve impulses, muscle reflexes and energy levels. This move is an exercise of delicate precision requiring full concentration on the part of the Bowen therapist. To allow for even pressure throughout the Bowen move, there are no fast or jerky movements, but a smooth rolling motion over the body structure. The roll over the nerve, muscle, tendon or ligament is performed with light to medium pressure and ensures if performed correctly, consistent and even pressure

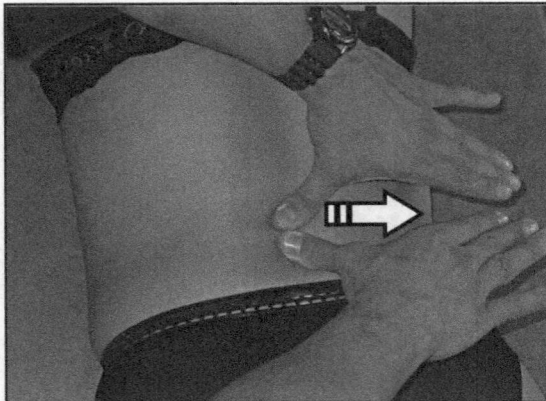

throughout the complete move itself. Pressure is usually transferred from the tips of the thumbs or fingers to the belly or pads of the thumbs or fingers in a rolling action. The Bowen move should not be painful for the client, though there may be instances where sensitivity can be found in some individuals. For this reason it is important to get feedback throughout the procedure from the client. Performing the Bowen move also allows the Bowen therapist to monitor muscle tension and to allow comparison from one side of the body to the other.

The skilled Bowen therapist will make this move look very easy but behind its wonderful simple appearance, lies an intricate complexity as well as an amazing chain of events that occurs when it performs its work on the human body.

Procedures or sequences

A series of Bowen moves on different areas of the body makes up a specific procedure. Although even one Bowen move can be very effective, performing the moves in a specific series has much greater benefits for the healing process within the body. There are a number of different Bowen procedures that can be performed both by themselves or in combination to assist a variety of different health problems. The Bowen therapist is trained to perform all of these procedures. Generally, fewer procedures are performed on your first visit to prepare the body to adjust to the changes and then gradually more procedures are added depending on the type of health condition or how chronic the problems are. The maximum number of times that one specific procedure is performed on the same day is two. These procedures and their applications will all be discussed in greater detail in the following chapter.

Two-minute breaks

As briefly mentioned earlier, throughout many of the Bowen procedures there are short two-minute breaks (in some procedures there are even longer breaks required) that are an important aspect of the Bowen method. These breaks after a series of moves allow the body to decipher the information that has been transferred by the stimulus to the nerves and other body structures. The Bowen method should not be rushed and these periodic breaks are necessary to achieve its full benefits. You may find that your Bowen therapist will even leave the room during this time and it is not because he or she is sneaking away for a break but to allow the energy channels in your body to balance and messages sent to the brain to be deciphered and redistributed to areas of the body.

Breathing

In many cases during the application of the Bowen moves, your therapist will ask you to slowly inhale and then exhale, especially when doing moves on the chest, upper back or abdominal area. As you are inhaling, they will be pulling back the skin slack as in Part 1 of the Bowen move, then they will apply light pressure and ask you to exhale. As you are exhaling, part 3 of the Bowen move is performed. This method allows the Bowen move to be performed without any interference or resistance due to breathing and ensures the highest degree of safety. The principle is the same as when we exercise or contract a muscle when lifting a weight. We learn to breathe out when we lift or perform the exercise and to breathe in when we relax.

The basis of the Bowen method is the Bowen move. Its design by Tom Bowen is wonderfully simple, its application beautifully elegant, its benefits far-reaching and its effectiveness pleasantly surprising. It serves to remind us once again that the most effective methods do not have to be complicated, as modern medicine often would like us to believe. Simple as the Bowen move may appear, the chain of events that are triggered in the body after its gentle light touch have baffled even the greatest scientific minds of today. Just as the cell is the basic unit of life for the body, the Bowen move is the basic unit of each of the Bowen procedures, which will be explained in the next chapter.

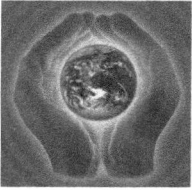

Fundamental Bowen procedures

13

This chapter will give you an idea of the range of fundamental procedures that are used in Bowen therapy. As mentioned before the explanations are not designed as a guide on how to perform Bowen but as a general overview of what is performed during each procedure. Please note that this is not a complete manual on how to perform the Bowen method. Those who wish to learn the Bowen method are strongly advised to take a course as practical sessions are necessary in order to correctly locate points and to effectively perform the moves safely.

For each procedure there is a short overview and a short explanation of each move in the sequence. A few samples of photographs of some locations of the moves are included, as well as some anatomical locations to give you an idea of how the procedure is performed. Health problems that may be assisted by the procedure as well as any special comments pertaining to each are noted.

1. Lower Back Procedure

This procedure is the first part of three procedures that are often called the basic or relaxation moves. Most clients will receive these three procedures on their first visit and they often form prerequisites for other procedures. They are the basic moves that work holistically on the whole body, that release general muscle tension and prepare the body for other moves. Most work performed by Bowen therapists centers around these important 3 procedures. As these procedures work across all meridians of the body, they have been known to address a wide range of health problems. On especially the first visit, I usually recommend all three relaxation procedures be performed to prepare the client for further specific procedures.

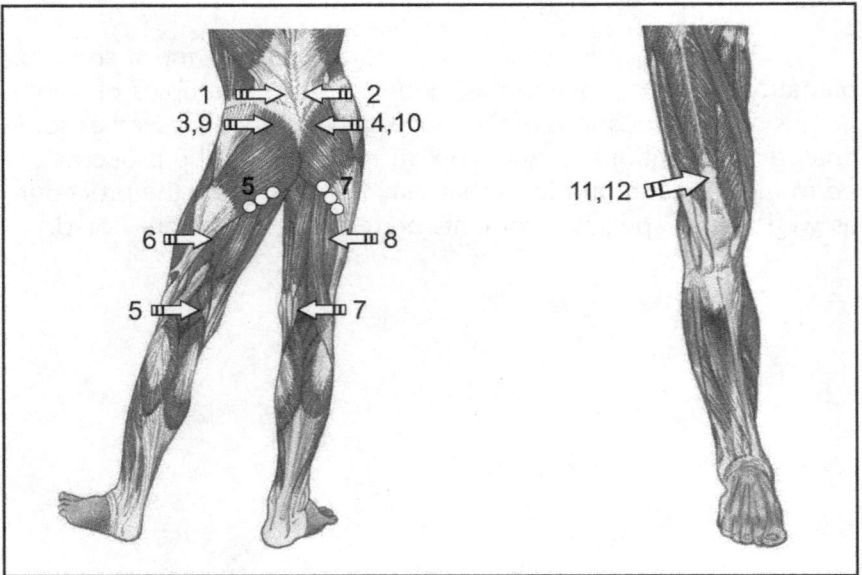

Preparation: The client lies on their stomach, hands by their side and head turned to the side. Most procedures begin on the left side of the client as in Bowen therapy the left side is considered the negative side, which acts as an "earth" and the right side is considered the positive side of the body.

The first two moves act to contain or block the energy and impulses to only the lower part of the body and for this reason they are often called "stoppers" or "blockers."

Move 1:

The therapist places both thumbs on the **left erector spinae** muscle, two finger widths above the **iliac crest** and moves the skin in the lateral direction (away from the midline of the body), applies gentle pressure on the lateral side of the erector spinae muscle, holds for a few seconds and then applies a Bowen move in the medial direction (towards the midline of the body) applying constant pressure.

Move 2:

The therapist places both index fingers on the right erector spinae muscle, two finger widths above the iliac crest and moves the skin in the lateral direction, applies gentle pressure on the lateral side of the erector spinae muscle, holds for a few seconds and then applies a Bowen move in the medial direction applying constant pressure.

Move 3:

The therapist places both thumbs on the midpoint of the upper edge of the **gluteus maximus** muscle. The skin is drawn back laterally across the upper edge of the muscle, then firm pressure is applied, then returning medially with a rolling move across the upper edge of the gluteus maximus.

The therapist stands on right side of the client.

Move 4:

Same as in Move 3 except on the right side of the client.

Two minute pause (These pauses are designed to allow the body time to react to the moves)

Therapist stands on the left of the client.

The next move utilizes a holding point, which is a location where pressure is applied to redirect the move that is being applied at the same time. It is similar to the "stoppers" except that it lasts only as long as pressure is being applied.

Move 5:

The therapist places the fingers of the left hand at the midpoint of the **gluteal crease** or fold, and firmly applies and maintains pressure. The right thumb is placed across the fibers of the short head of the **biceps femoris** muscle just above the **popliteal fossa** (back of the knee). The skin is drawn back laterally, a short pause and then a move with firmer pressure is applied returning to the starting point. If the move is properly administered, an impulse can be felt at the holding point. The therapist removes both hands.

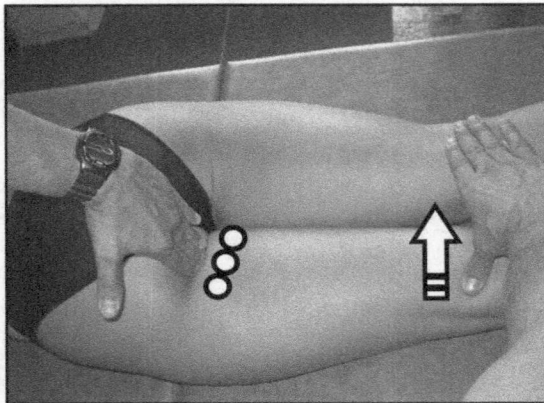

Move 6:

The therapist places both thumbs on the midpoint of the **vastus lateralis** muscle. The skin is drawn down anteriorly (towards the front part of the body) and then a Bowen move with gently pressure is administered upwards or posteriorly (towards the back of the body).

The therapist stands on the right side of the client.

Move 7:

This move is the same holding point as in Move 5, except the therapist applies and maintains pressure with the fingers of the right hand. The move across the fibers of the **biceps femoris** muscle is made using the left thumb. If the move is properly administered, an impulse can be felt at the holding point. The therapist removes both hands.

Move 8:

This move is the same as Move 6 except on the right side.

Two minute pause.

Move 9:

Repeat Move 3.

Move 10:

Repeat Move 4.

Turn the client on their back.

Move 11:

The therapist places both thumbs under the lateral border of the tendon of the **vastus lateralis** muscle approximately 2 cm (1 inch) proximal (towards the head) to the patella. The skin slack is drawn back down. The thumbs firmly apply pressure while the move is slowly made upwards and medially until they pluck across the tendon.

The therapist stands on the client's right side.

Move 12:

Same as in Move 11, except on the right side of the client.

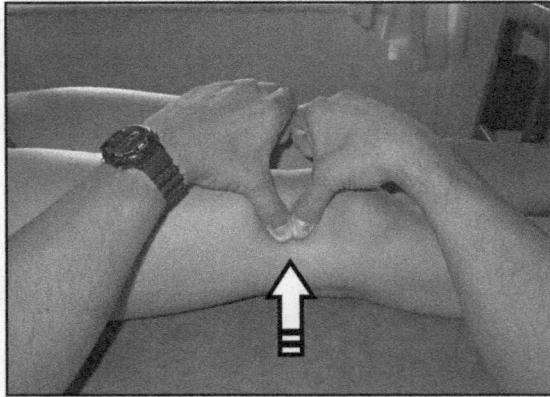

Health Problems that may be assisted

- Lower back pain

- Body relaxation

- Muscle tension release and balance

- Ischias pain

- Arthritis

- Adrenal gland

- Blood pressure problems

- Constipation

- Edema in the lower part of the body

- Lymphatic drainage

- Leg cramps

- Liver disease

- Menopause, menstrual difficulties

- Osteoporosis

- Lower back pain during pregnancy

- Skin problems

- Varicose veins

- Flow of energy

- Detoxification

- Stress

Special Comments

This procedure can also be performed in a sitting position or on the side if the client is unable to lay flat or on the stomach (as in pregnancy, injuries, deformities).

2. Upper and mid-back procedure

This procedure is the second of the relaxation moves and usually follows the lower back procedure. It is also a prerequisite for other procedures. It addresses the upper back, middle back, scapula and the shoulders.

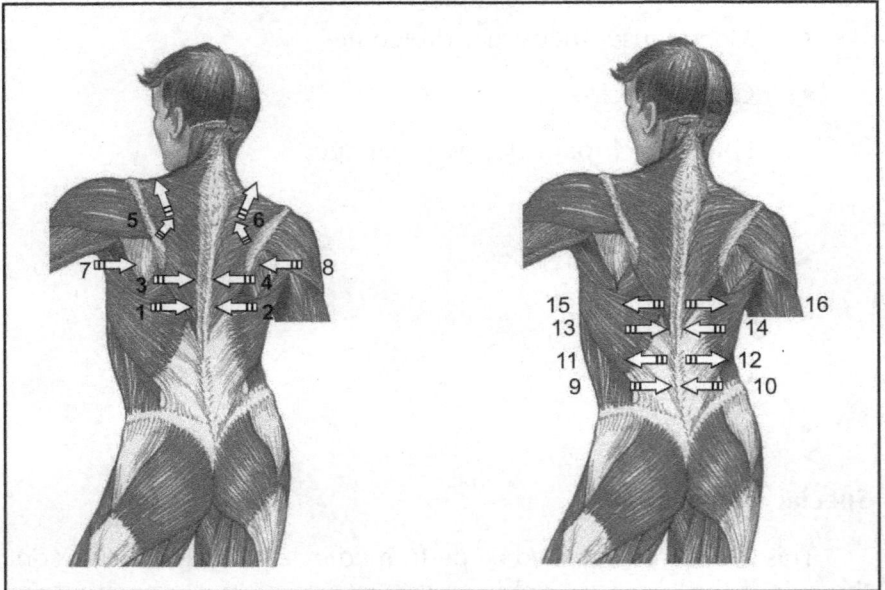

Prerequisite: Lower back procedure

Preparation: The client lies on their back, hands by their sides and head turned to the side. The therapist stands on the client's left side.

The first four moves are performed around the lower part of the scapula. They are similar to the first two moves performed in the lower back procedure and they are also considered "stoppers" or "blockers" and they ensure that the impulses remain in the upper back area.

84

Moves 1 to 4 are performed at the same time as the client exhales.

Move 1:

The therapist places both thumbs just below the lower edge of the left scapula on the left **erector spinae** muscle. The skin is drawn back laterally, and a Bowen move is applied across the erector spinae muscle in the medial direction.

Move 2:

This move is the same as Move 1 except using both index fingers on the right erector spinae muscle. The therapist moves the skin back laterally and then applies the Bowen move in the medial direction.

Move 3:

This move is the same as Move 1 except two finger widths upwards (superior).

Move 4:

This move is the same as Move 2 except two finger widths upwards (superior).

Two minute pause.

The client turns their head over to the side away from the therapist.

Move 5:

The therapist places the thumb of their left hand approximately one third of the distance down from the upper edge of the left scapula. The index finger of the right hand is placed so that the tip is touching the tip of the left thumb. Both thumb and index finger move together drawing the skin back inferiorly and then a move is made in a semi-circle across the **rhomboideus major** muscle. The thumb is lifted, and the index finger remains and moves the skin back. The thumb is placed back in position and this time pressure is applied and a rolling move is made across the **rhomboideus minor** muscle and the **levator scapula** muscle.

The therapist moves to the right side of the client.

Client turns their head on the side away from the therapist.

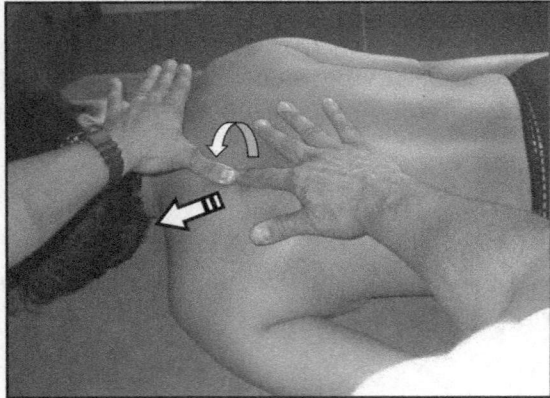

Move 6:

This move is the same as Move 5 but on the right side of the client.

Two minute pause.

Move 7:

The therapist places both thumbs on the lateral edge of the **latissimus dorsi** muscle in line with the lower border of the scapula. The skin slack is moved down and then the move is made upwards and medially.

The therapist moves to the right side of the client.

Move 8:

This move is the same as Move 7 but on the right side of the client.

Two minute pause.

The therapist moves to the left side of the client.

Moves 9 to 16 are made during exhalation. The area between the lower edge of the scapula and the upper edge of the iliac crest is divided into quarters.

Move 9:

The therapist places both thumbs 2 cm (1 inch) above the iliac crests on the left erector spinae muscle. The skin slack is moved back in the lateral direction and then a medial Bowen move is made across the erector spinae muscle.

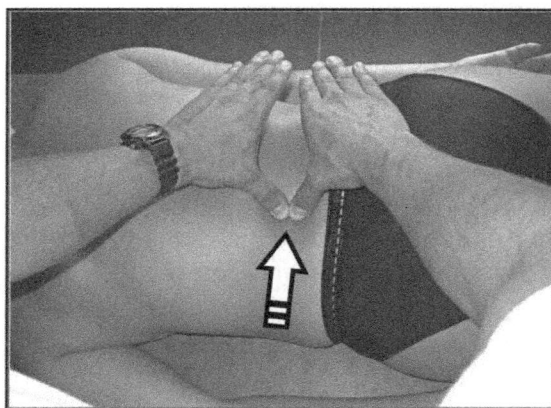

Move 10:

The therapist places both index fingers and places them on the right erector spinae muscle on the opposite side of Move 9. The skin slack is moved back laterally and then a medial Bowen move is made across the erector spinae muscle.

Move 11:

The therapist places either thumbs or index fingers a quarter distance up from (superior to) Move 9 on the left erector spinae muscle. The skin slack is moved back medially and then a lateral Bowen move is performed across the left erector spinae muscle.

Move 12:

The therapist places both thumbs opposite to Move 11 on the right erector spinae muscle. The skin slack is moved back medially and then a lateral Bowen move is performed across the right erector spinae muscle.

Move 13:

This move is the same as Move 9 except one-quarter distance up on the left erector spinae muscle.

Move 14:

This move is the same as Move 10, except one-quarter distance up on the right erector spinae muscle.

Move 15:

This move is the same as Move 11, except one-quarter distance up on the left erector spinae muscle.

Move 16:

This move is the same as Move 12, except one-quarter distance up on the right erector spinae muscle.

Health Problems that may be assisted

- Lower back pain
- Body relaxation
- Cervical to thoracic spine problems
- Pressure around the scapula
- Arthritis
- Shoulder pain
- Breathing difficulties
- Energy flow
- Detoxification
- Muscle tension balance
- Asthma
- Scoliosis
- Lymphatic drainage

Special Comments

This procedure can also be performed in a sitting position or on the side if the client is unable to lay flat or on the stomach (as in pregnancy, injuries, deformities).

3. Neck and shoulders procedure

This procedure is the third of the relaxation moves and usually follows the upper and mid-back procedure. It is also a prerequisite for other procedures. It addresses the neck, upper back and shoulders.

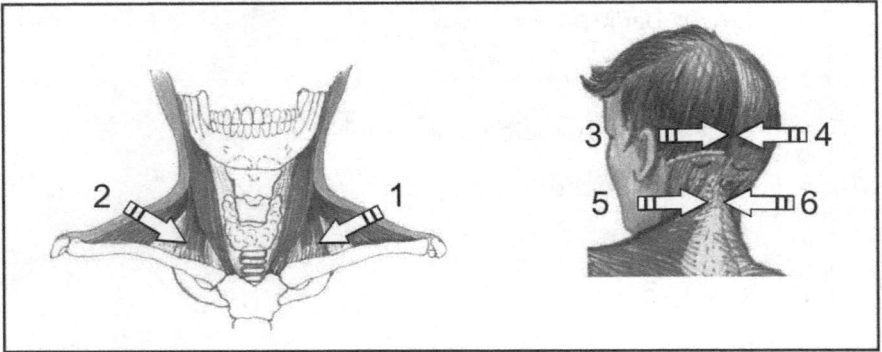

Prerequisite: Upper and mid-back procedure

Preparation: The client lies on their back, hands by their sides. The therapist stands at the head of the client.

Move 1:

The therapist places their left thumb into the hollow beside the lateral borders of the **scalenus** muscles. The move is made upwards and medially across the scalenus muscles.

Move 2:

This move is the same as Move 1 except on the right side using the right thumb.

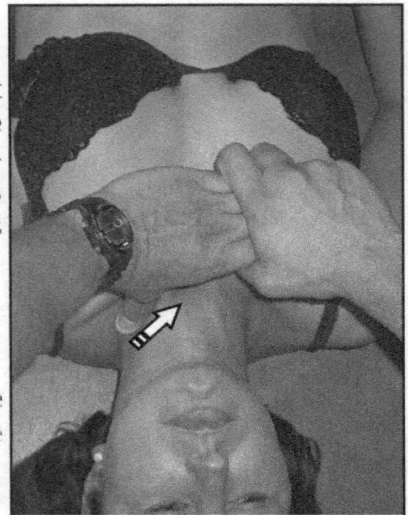

Move 3:

The therapist places their hands behind the client's head, palms facing upwards and places the left middle finger over the left **semi-spinalis capitus** muscle, inferiolateral (1 finger width down and 1 finger width to the side) to the occipital condyle. The skin slack is moved laterally and then a gently move is made in the medial direction across the belly of the semispinalis capitus.

Move 4:

This move is the same as Move 3, except on the right side using the right middle finger.

Two minute pause.

Move 5:

The therapist places their hands behind the client's neck, palms facing upwards and places the middle finger of the left hand on the left **trapezius** muscle. The skin is moved laterally and then pressure is applied on the trapezius while at the same time moving slowly medially.

Move 6:

This move is the same as Move 5, except on the right side using the right middle finger.

Two minute pause.

Repeat Moves 5 and 6.

Two minute pause.

If muscle release is not achieved it may be necessary to repeat Moves 1 to 6.

Health Problems that may be assisted

- Pain or problems in the neck to shoulder area

- Body relaxation

- Neck pain

- Migraines or headaches

- Muscle tension balance

- Energy flow

- Detoxification

- Lymphatic Drainage

- Stress

- Whiplash injuries

Special Comments

All neck moves should be performed gently and very slowly.

4. Upper Respiratory and Temporomandibular joint procedure

This procedure addresses the upper respiratory passages, provides excellent lymphatic drainage for the head and sinus area and balances the upper back, neck and jaw.

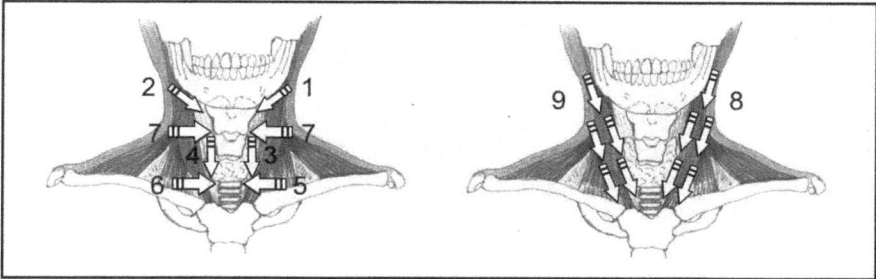

Prerequisite: Moves 1 to 8 of the Upper and mid-back procedure and Moves 1 to 6 of the Neck and shoulders procedure

Preparation: The client lies on their back, hands by their sides. The therapist stands behind the head of the client.

Move 1:

The therapist places their left index or middle finger on the midpoint of the left mandible. The skin slack is taken back towards the angle of the mandible and a gentle move is made forwards.

Move 2:

This move is the same as Move 1, except on the right side, using the right index or middle finger.

Move 3:

The therapist places their left index or middle finger on the midpoint between the chin and the clavicle on the left lateral aspect of the thyroid cartilage at the level of the Adam's apple. The skin slack is moved upwards (superiorly) and a gentle move is made downwards (inferiorly)

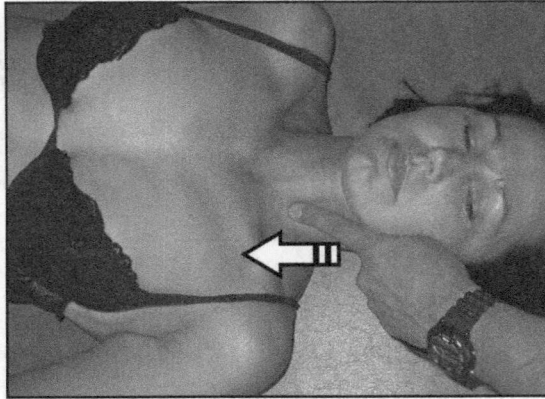

Move 4:

This move is the same as Move 3, except on the right side using the right index or middle finger.

Move 5:

The therapist places the index finger of the left hand on the **sternocleidomastoid** muscle where it attaches to the sternum about 2 cm (1 inch) up from the left clavicle. The skin slack is moved back laterally and then a medial move is made using only medium pressure.

Move 6:

This move is the same as Move 5, except on the right side using the right index finger.

Move 7:

The therapist places both middle fingers of both hands on both lateral sides of the trachea. The trachea is gently moved from side to side twice.

Move 8:

The therapist applies a series of moves using a pinching pressure on the left sternocleidomastoid muscle with the thumb and index finger. The moves begin just above where the sternocleidomastoid muscle attaches to the sternum and move progressively upwards towards the mastoid process. The skin slack is drawn upwards and then pressure is applied with the thumb and index finger in a downward direction. This is repeated many times. Once reaching the mastoid process, the series of moves is completed by drawing the skin back upwards (superiorly) with the thumb or index finger and making a firm move downwards (inferiorly) over the fibers of the sternocleidomastoid at the mastoid process.

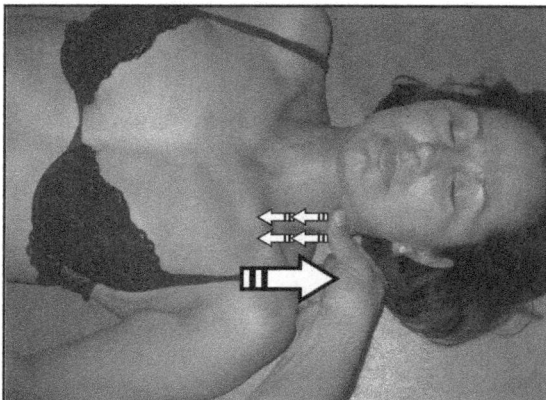

Move 9:

This series of moves is the same as Move 8, except on the right side.

Moves 8 and 9 can be repeated up to three times if the lymph nodes are tender. A five-minute pause is left between each of these series of moves.

The therapist now asks the client to place the knuckle of their index finger between their teeth and to relax the jaw.

Move 10:

The therapist places their left index finger on the left side of the client's head and moves the skin slack back forward (anteriorly) and makes a gentle move back (posteriorly) over the condylar fossa.

Move 11:

The therapist maintains position as in Move 10 and using their left index finger, moves the skin superiorly and then makes a gentle move inferiorly over the condylar fossa.

Move 12:

This move is the same as Move 10, except over the right condylar fossa using the right index finger.

Move 13:

This move is the same as Move 11, except over the right condylar fossa using the right index finger.

Move 14:

The therapist places their left index finger on the left midpoint of the posterior border of the mandible. The skin slack is moved upwards (superiorly) and then a gentle move is made downwards (inferiorly).

Move 15:

This move is the same as Move 14, except on the right side using the right index finger.

Move 16:

The therapist places their left index finger or middle finger anterior to the top of the ear and superior to the zygomatic process. The skin slack is moved upwards in the anterior direction and then a gentle move is made downwards (posteriorly).

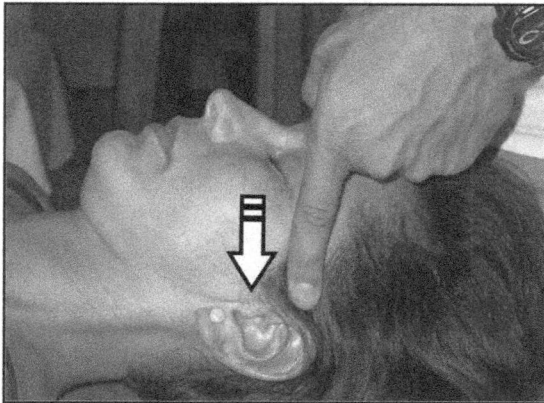

Move 17:

This move is the same as Move 16, except on the right side using the right index or middle finger.

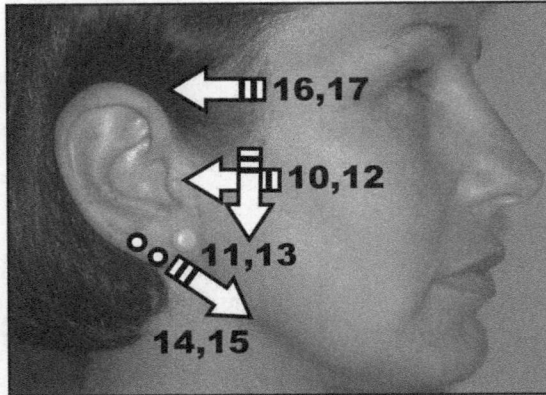

Health Problems that may be assisted

- Lymphatic drainage

- Migraines and headaches

- Upper respiratory breathing difficulties

- Allergies, hay fever

- Asthma

- Tinnitus

- Ear infections

- Vision problems

- Colds, flu, sore throats and congested sinuses

- Jaw problems

- Grinding teeth or clicking in the jaw
- Facial nerve paralysis
- Stress

Special Comments

There may be a chance of some changes in the jaw, which may affect the bite. Those with extensive dental restoration should be advised of this possibility.

Excessive opening of the mouth should be avoided for a few days after this procedure.

5. Knee procedure

This procedure addresses the knee, which is often prone to injury, swelling and cramping and is also excellent for lymphatic drainage. It allows fluid to drain from the knee and promotes better healing. It also relieves tension that often causes lower back pain so it can be combined together with the lower back procedures for beneficial results.

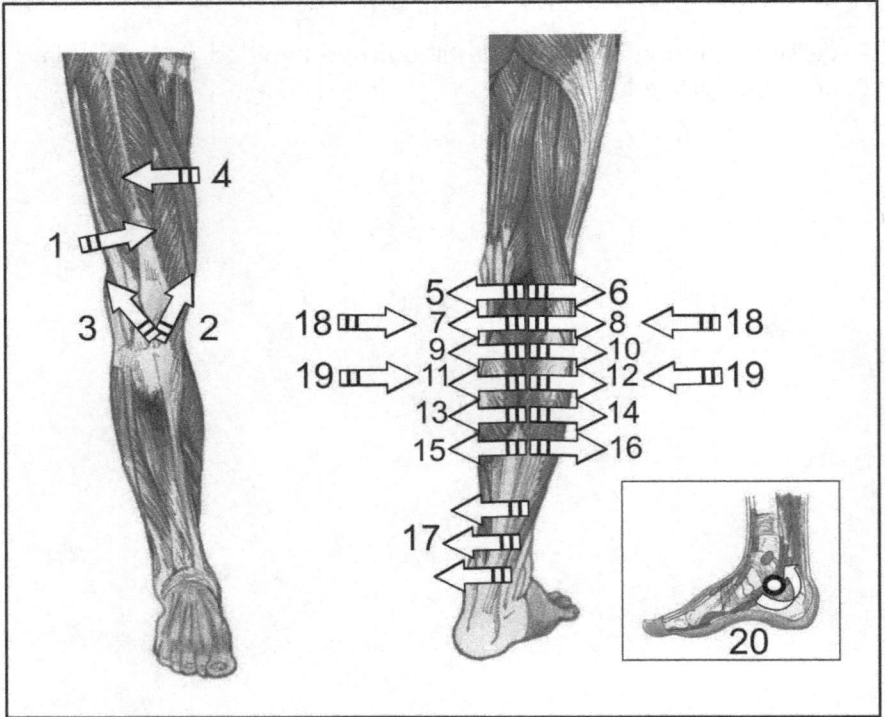

Prerequisite: Lower back procedure

Preparation: Client is placed on their back and the therapist stands on the client's left side.

Move 1:

The therapist places both thumbs under the lateral border of the tendon of the vastus lateralis muscle approximately 2 cm (1 inch) proximal (towards the head) to the patella. The skin slack is drawn back down. The thumbs firmly apply pressure while the move is slowly made upwards and medially until they pluck across the tendon.

Move 2:

The therapist using their index finger makes an oblique medial move over the retinacular fibers over the medial femoral condyle near the middle aspect of the patella.

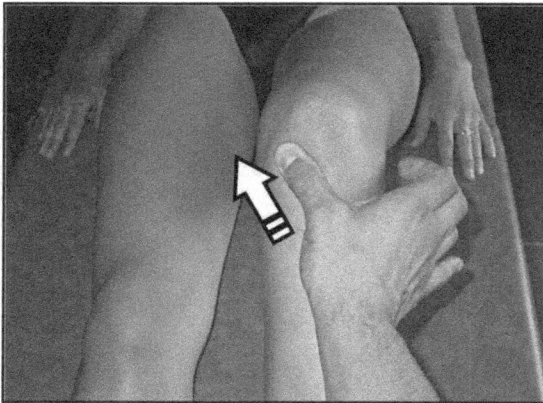

Move 3:

The therapist using their thumb makes an oblique lateral move over the retinacular fibers over the lateral femoral condyle near the middle aspect of the patella.

Two-minute pause.

Move 4:

The therapist places both their index fingers about 3 to 4 finger widths superior to the patella and makes a lateral move over the **vastus medialis** muscle.

Bend the client's knee to 90 degrees.

Move 5 and 6:

The therapist places the fingers of both their hands over the medial and lateral heads of the **gastrocnemius** about 4 cm (1.5 - 2 inches) below the point of insertion of the hamstrings. The two muscle heads of the gastrocnemius muscle are separated using first a medial and then a lateral move.

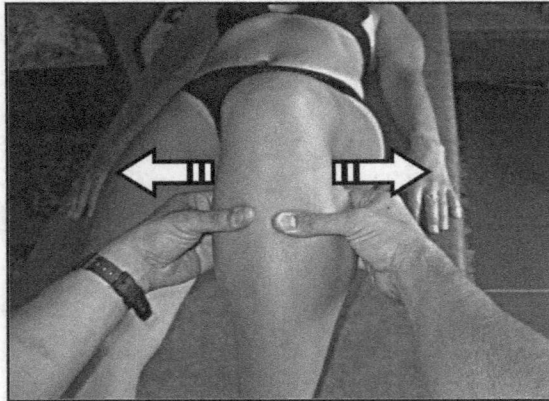

Two-minute pause.

Moves 7 to 16:

The therapist progresses down the leg (distally) from the position of Moves 5 and 6 and gently separates the gastrocnemius muscle by alternating medial and lateral moves, until just before the Achilles tendon.

Move 17:

The therapist performs three medial moves 1 cm (0.5 inches) apart, from the proximal to the distal end of the Achilles tendon.

Two-minute pause.

Moves 18 and 19:

The therapist uses both hands linked together and closes both heads of the gastrocnemius together with gentle pressure. Move 18 is applied over the upper belly of the muscle and Move 19 is applied over the lower aspect.

Move 20:

The therapist places the thumb or index finger posterior to the medial maleolus of the ankle and moves the skin slack down towards the heel and makes a move up and around the medial maleolus, moving the tibial nerve and neurovascular bundle.

Health Problems that may be assisted

- Any knee problem
- Lymphatic drainage
- Edema
- Varicose veins
- Lower back pain
- Ankle problems
- Kidney or liver problems
- Cramps in the legs

Special Comments

Avoid exercise for at least a week after the Bowen session. Avoid bending or squatting right after for at least 24 hours.

6. Frozen shoulder procedure

This procedure addresses the shoulder and rotator cuff and includes a simple series of extremely effective moves that often release tension immediately after application. I have witnessed many times that some clients with frozen shoulder can immediately raise their arm right after this procedure. Injuries to the shoulder can be extremely difficult to heal and clients can often complain of pain in the area when there is any kind of movement. In a high percentage

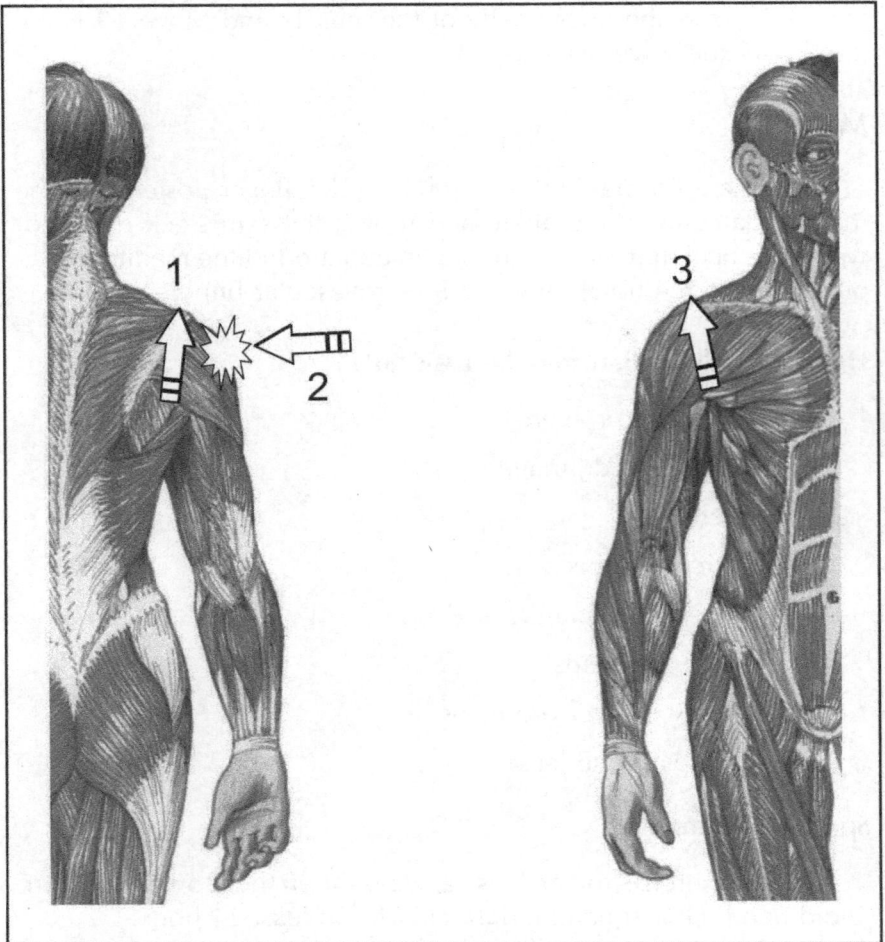

of cases after only three Bowen sessions and specific prescribed exercises, pain and swelling often disappear and free movement is restored to the rotator cuff area. This procedure is also effective for any breathing problems or asthma as it relieves tension so that the upper chest can freely expand.

Prerequisite: Moves 1 to 8 of the Upper and mid-back procedure and Moves 1 to 6 of the Neck and shoulder procedure

Preparation: The client sits in a chair or on the massage table. The therapist stands facing the client's face, always applying the procedure to both arms, starting with the better shoulder first. The therapist holds and supports the client's left elbow using their left hand and places their right leg between the client's knees.

Move 1:

The therapist moves the client's left elbow in the direction of the right shoulder while at the same time makes a move with both middle fingers over the lower border of the posterior **deltoid** muscle upwards (superiorly). The therapist should feel a vibration or impulse at the triceps area above the client's elbow. If it is not felt, repeat the move again.

Move 2:

The therapist maintains the client's left elbow in a point of maximal adduction and hits the lateral aspect of the left shoulder with the heel of the right hand. The therapist then returns the client's arm to the starting position.

Move 3:

The therapist makes a move using their right thumb across the lower fibers of the anterior deltoid in the superior direction.

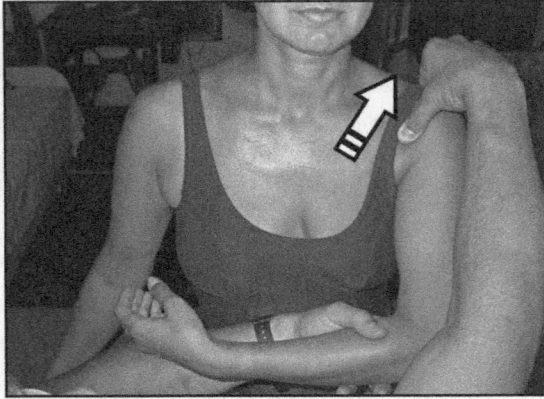

Repeat Moves 1 to 3 on the other shoulder.

This procedure is repeated after 7 days and then again only after 4 weeks.

Health Problems that may be assisted

- Any shoulder problems
- Frozen shoulder or reduced movement in the shoulder joint or arm
- Asthma or breathing difficulties
- Rotator cuff injuries

Special Comments

Special exercises for the shoulder are prescribed after the Bowen session. Allow 4 weeks after the second Bowen session to allow the shoulder to allow the area to heal itself before the next session.

7. Respiratory Procedure

This procedure addresses the respiratory system. It is used for any respiratory problems including asthma, bronchitis, emphysema, chest pain and other ailments as well as any heart complaints. It is also quite effective for digestive complaints, stimulating the liver, pancreas and gall bladder.

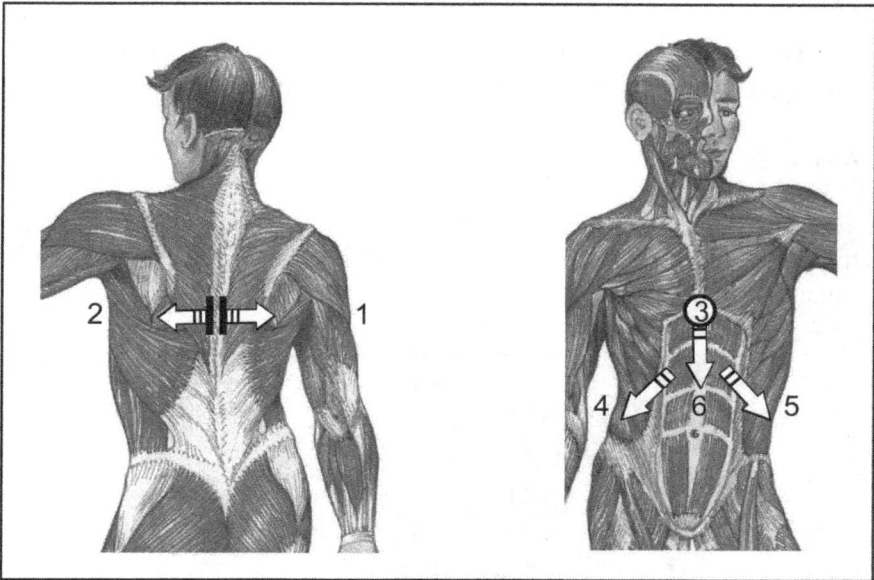

Prerequisite: Moves 1 to 8 of the Upper and mid-back procedure

Preparation: Place the client on their stomach, head turned to the left. The therapist stands on the client's left side.

Move 1:

The therapist, using their right hand, flexes the client's left knee to 90 degrees and then moves the leg laterally as far as possible within comfort levels and holds it steady in that position. The therapist then places the fingers of their left hand over the right **iliocostalis** muscle just above the lower aspect of the scapula. On the client's inspiration, the skin slack is drawn back medially and on expiration a lateral move is made across the iliocostalis muscle.

The client is asked to turn their head to the right side. The therapist stands by the right side of the client.

Move 2:

This move is the same as Move 1, except on the right side and the move is made with the opposite hand over the left iliocostalis muscle.

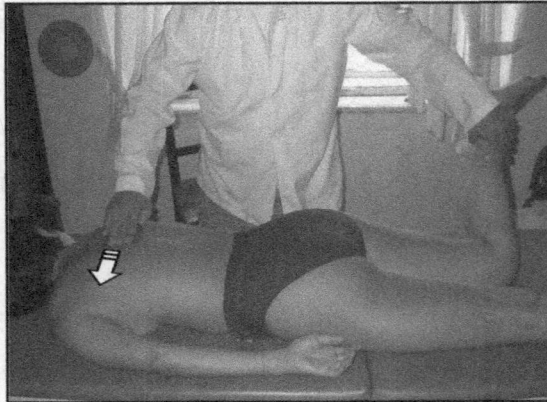

Two-minute pause.

The client turns over onto their back. The therapist stands by the left side of the client.

Move 3:

Move 3 is a holding point.

The therapist gently applies pressure using their right thumb or middle finger to the epigastrium, just below the xyphoid process. This point is held while Moves 4 and 5 are performed.

Move 4:

On the client's complete exhalation, the therapist, using their left thumb, makes a lateral oblique move at the midpoint of the lower border of the left rib cage, across the left **rectus abdominis** muscle.

Move 5:

On the client's complete exhalation, the therapist, using their left middle finger, makes a lateral oblique move at the midpoint of the lower border of the right rib cage, across the right rectus abdominis muscle.

Move 6:

The therapist releases their right hand and the holding point from Move 3 and places their left middle finger just below the holding point in Move 3. The skin slack is drawn upwards (superiorly) and a gently move is made downwards (inferiorly) across the rectus abdominis muscle.

Health Problems that may be assisted

- Any breathing difficulties

- Asthma

- Allergies and colds

- Bronchitis

- Hernia
- Stomach or digestive problems
- Heartburn
- Liver, pancreas and gall bladder problems
- Nausea
- Colicky infants

Special Comments

Variations of this procedure can be used during an asthma attack but medical attention should still be obtained.

8. Hamstring procedure

This procedure addresses the hamstring area and is particularly useful for sporting injuries. It is also used to complement the knee or pelvic procedure for difficult or stubborn conditions.

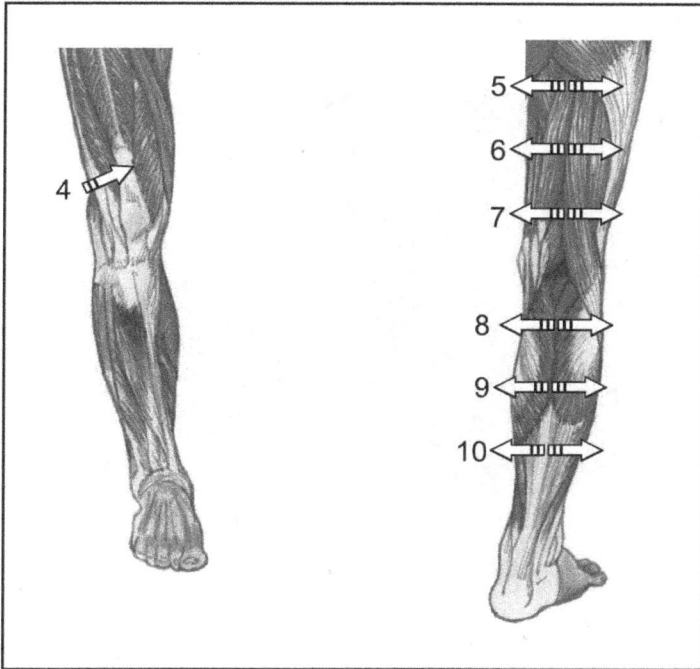

Prerequisite: Moves 1 to 8 of the Lower back procedure

Preparation: The client lies on their stomach, the therapist stands on the client's left side, facing the legs.

Move 1:

The therapist, using their right hand, flexes the client's left knee to 90 degrees, in order to relax the **hamstring** and **biceps femoris** muscles. The therapist then places their fingers or elbow on the midpoint of the gluteal crease or fold and applies deep pressure. The skin slack is drawn back laterally and with firm pressure a medial move is performed.

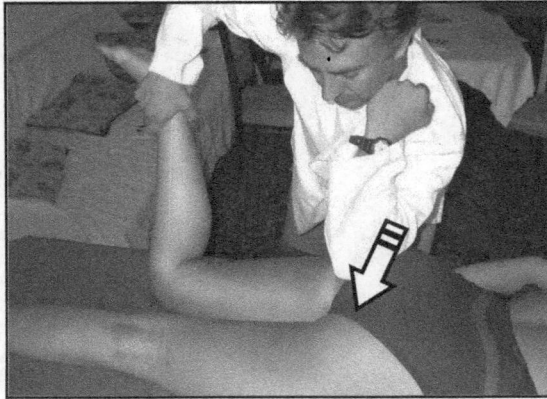

Move 2:

The therapist holds the leg at 90 degrees as in Move 1 and places their thumb in the middle of the popliteal fossa approximately 2 cm (1 inch) above the skin crease. The skin slack is drawn back laterally and a gentle move is made in the medial direction.

Move 3:

The therapist holds the leg just below the ankle with their left hand while at the same time their right hand holds the client's foot and toes. The foot is rotated for a few seconds in the clockwise and counter-clockwise directions. The move is completed by striking the sole of the foot across the third metatarsal.

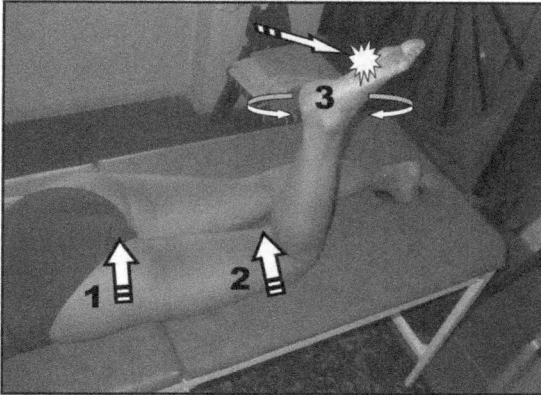

Repeat Moves 1 to 3 on the right side, then client turns over onto their back.

Five-minute pause.

Move 4:

The therapist places both thumbs under the lateral border of the tendon of the **vastus lateralis** muscle approximately 2 cm (1 inch) proximal (towards the head) to the patella. The skin slack is drawn back down. The thumbs firmly apply pressure while the move is slowly made upwards and medially until they pluck across the tendon.

If this move evokes pain or tenderness, administrate Moves 2 to 4 of the Knee Procedure before continuing on.

Preparation for Moves 5 to 9:

The client's knee is flexed to 90 degrees and the therapist stands facing the client's feet. The therapist positions his hands with arms encircling the client's lower leg.

Move 5:

The therapist positions their fingers deep at the midpoint of the gluteal fold. The hand medial draws the skin slack back laterally and then performs a firm medial move over the hamstring and biceps femoris muscles. The hand lateral draws the skin slack back medially and then performs a firm lateral move.

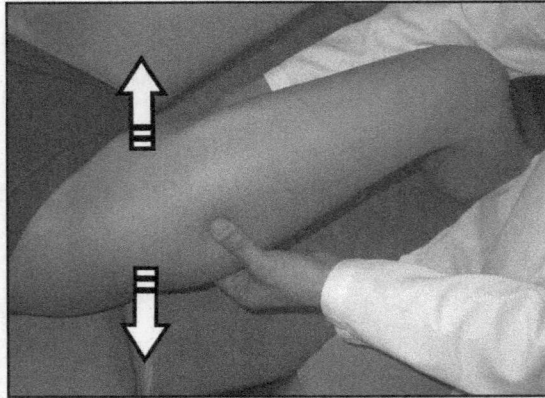

Move 6:

This move is the same as Move 5, except the hands are placed lower at the midpoint of the thigh. The therapist again applies a medial and then a lateral move.

Move 7:

This move is the same as Move 5, except the hands are placed lower just above the middle of the popliteal fossa. The therapist again applies a medial and then a lateral move.

Move 8:

This move is the same as Move 5, except the hands are placed lower below the knee over the medial and lateral heads of the gastrocnemius muscle approximately 4 cm (1.5 inches) below the insertion point of the tendons of the hamstrings. The therapist applies a medial and then a lateral move.

Move 9:

This move is the same as Move 5, except the hands are placed lower at the middle of the gastrocnemius muscle. The therapist applies a medial and then a lateral move.

Move 10:

This move is the same as Move 5, except the hands are placed lower over the Achilles' tendon. The therapist applies a medial and then a lateral move.

Repeat Moves 4 to 10 on the right leg.

Health Problems that may be assisted

- Injury or tension in the hamstrings
- Cramps
- Varicose veins
- For knee problems to support the knee procedure
- For the pelvis to support the pelvic procedure

Special Comments

Hamstring stretching exercises are recommended after the Bowen session.

9. Pelvic procedure

This procedure addresses the pelvis and is also used for uneven leg length discrepancies as well as for lymphatic drainage. Surprisingly, it is also effective for fever conditions such as the flu and can be used as a complement procedure for stubborn lower back conditions.

Prerequisite: Moves 1 to 8 of the Lower back procedure with client lying on their stomach

Preparation: The client lies on their back.

Move 1:

The therapist places both thumbs under the lateral border of the tendon of the **vastus lateralis** muscle approximately 2 cm (1 inch) proximal (towards the head) to the patella. The skin slack is drawn back down. The thumbs firmly apply pressure while the move is slowly made upwards and medially until they pluck across the tendon.

Move 2:

The therapist flexes the hip and externally rotates the thigh in order to locate the **gracilis** and **adductor longus** muscles. Two fingers of each hand are placed below the gracilis muscle and then the leg is returned to its original position. The skin slack is drawn back down posteriorly and with firm pressure, this point is held for 20 seconds. During the last 10 seconds, the client is asked to take two slow and deep breaths and on complete exhalation of the second breath, a move is made upwards (anteriorly) across the gracilis muscle.

Move 3:

The therapist places both thumbs on the medial border of the **sartorius** muscle just below its origin. The skin slack is drawn back laterally and then with medium pressure a medial move is made over the sartorius muscle.

Move 4:

The therapist lifts the client's leg and moves it slightly laterally and then flexes the knee. The index finger of the upper hand is placed on the midpoint of the inguinal crease and the middle finger of the same hand is placed about 2.5 cm (1 inch) medial to it. The therapist's lower hand is placed on the front aspect of the client's flexed knee. The client is asked to inhale and then on exhalation, the therapist moves the client's knee in the direction of their opposite shoulder. At the same time the therapist applies a short move with the index and middle finger of their upper hand, moving superiorly. The therapist removes the upper hand in order to assist the client in extending the leg. The leg is then returned to its original resting position.

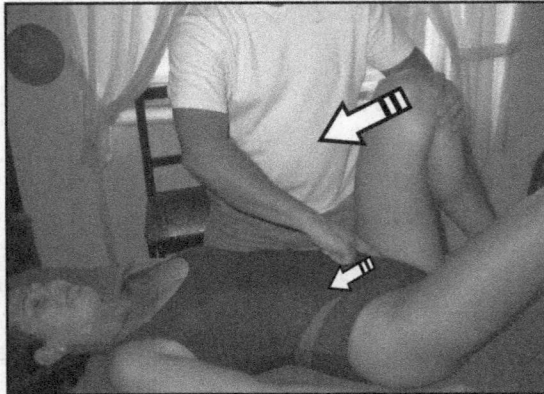

Moves 1 to 4 are then repeated on the other side.

Health Problems that may be assisted

- Any problems with the pelvis

- Poor body posture

- Uneven leg length

- Hernia

- Problems in the groin area

- Lower back pain

- Insufficient circulation

- Shin splints

- Any problems with the feet

- Fever

- Edema

- Groin tension

- Flu

- Lower leg cramps

- Varicose veins

Special Comments

Clients should not have their hip excessively moved as in Move 4 if they have undergone a hip replacement.

The area that is worked on is near the genitals and the client should be asked to cover the invasive area with their hands during the procedure. A test for groin tension is done before the procedure.

10. Coccyx procedure

This procedure is indicated for a variety of conditions and is truly a holistic sequence on its own. It addresses the reproductive system and assists in male and female infertility, improves urinary tract and prostate problems and is highly effective for stubborn migraine headaches. The coccyx is located at the base of the spine and this procedure promotes balance throughout the entire body, balancing all the chakras in the process. Many women who complain of premenstrual syndrome or menopausal symptoms find great relief after this procedure.

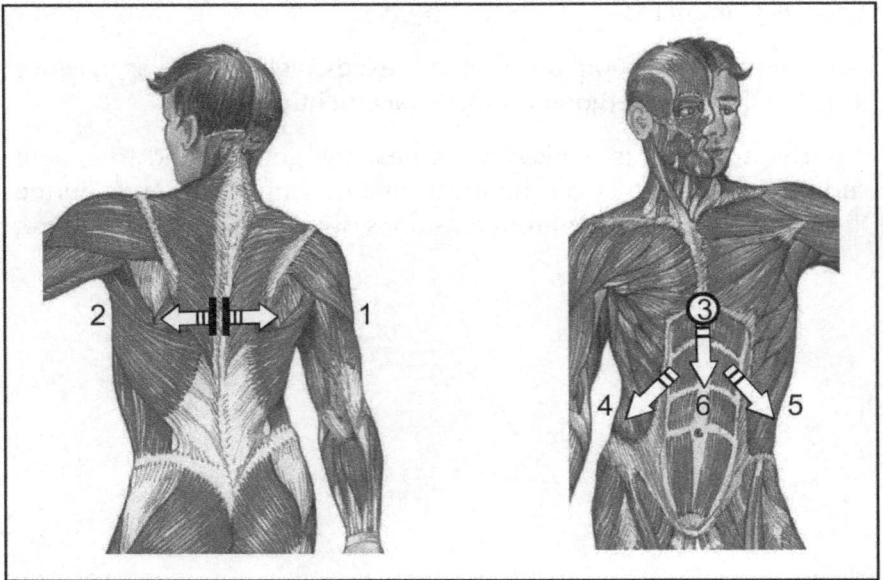

Prerequisite: Moves 1 to 8 of the Lower back procedure

Preparation: Gentle pressure is applied to either side of the coccyx to compare tenderness in the area. If neither side is tender, then the left side is treated.

The client is positioned on their stomach with their head turned to the left. The therapist stands at the left of the client. The left index finger is used to assess for tenderness. The following moves are explained for tenderness on the left side.

The Coccyx procedure is applied only on one side during a session.

Preparation for Move 1:

The therapist, using their right hand, flexes the client's left knee to 90 degrees and then moves the leg laterally as far as possible within comfort levels and holds it steady in that position.

The middle finger of their left hand is placed approximately 2.5 cm (1 inch) right of the natal cleft and palpates progressively down-wards until reaching the most inferior aspect of the sacrum. At this pont only soft tissue should be felt and the therapist firmly applies pressure with the middle finger. This is a holding point.

The index finger of the left hand is placed laterally on the left midpoint of the coccyx.

Move 1:

The therapist on the client's exhalation, performs a gentle move with the left index finger across the coccyx in the direction of the holding point.

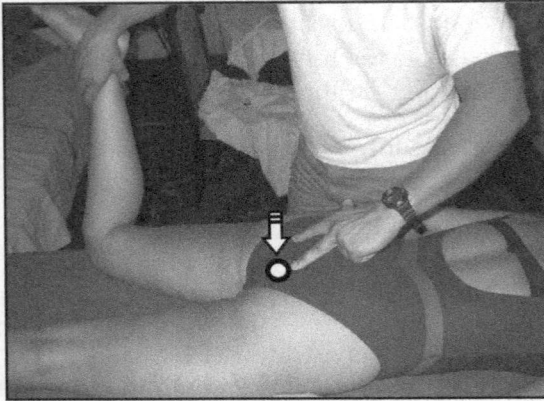

The client changes position to lying on their back with arms along their sides. The therapist stands at the left of the client.

Preparation for Move 2:

The therapist flexes the client's left knee to 90 degrees using their left hand. They then place their right middle finger on the midpoint of the line between the belly button and the midpoint of the inguinal ligament.

Move 2:

As the client inhales, the therapist draws the skin slack in the direction of the inguinal ligament with their right middle finger. On exhalation, a move is made across the lateral border of the left **rectus abdominus** muscle in the direction of the belly button and then laterally in the arc shape of a "boomerang." At the same time the client's left knee is moved in the direction of their opposite shoulder. The therapist then removes the right hand and uses both hands in order to assist the client in extending the leg. The leg is then returned to its original position.

Health Problems that may be assisted

- Migraines
- When one gluteal is lower than the other
- Bed-wetting in children
- Incontinence
- Any coccyx injuries
- Constipation or diarrhea
- Gynecological problems
- Premenstrual syndrome
- Menopausal symptoms
- Ovary or uterus problems
- Infertility
- Lower back pain
- Prostate problems
- Balance of chakras

Special Comments

The coccyx procedure is performed only on one side.

This procedure should not be used on pregnant women.

11. Kidney procedure

This procedure addresses the kidneys, which are often a weak area for many people in present times. Weak or insufficient kidney function can lead to a variety of problems including increased chance of infections, skin disease, chronic fatigue, fluctuations in blood pressure and migraine headaches.

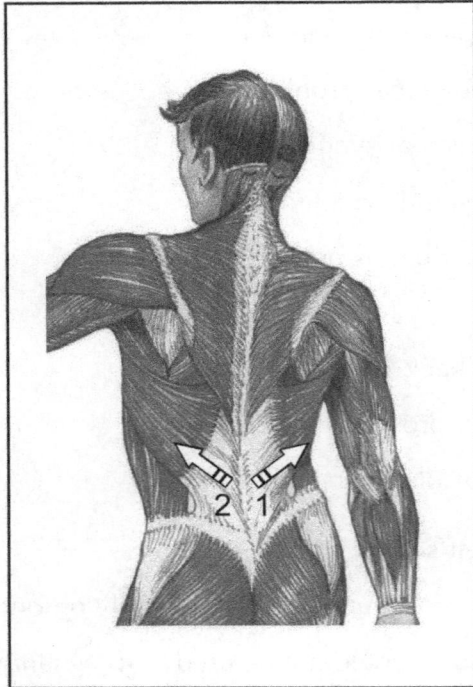

Prerequisite: Lower back procedure and Upper and mid-back procedure

Preparation: The client lies on their stomach, head turned to the left. The therapist stands on the client's left side.

Move 1:

The therapist uses their right hand to bend the client's left knee to 90 degrees, and then turns the leg laterally as far as possible within comfort. The leg is held in this position. The therapist places their left thumb below the lowest rib on the right erector spinae muscle. The skin slack is drawn medially and then an oblique move is made in the superiolateral direction across the right erector spinae muscle.

The client turns his head to the right; the therapist stands at the right of the client.

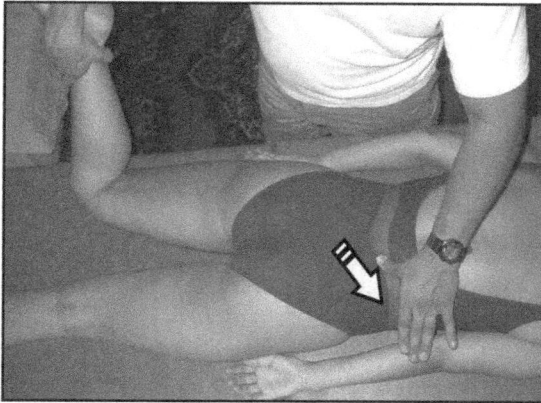

Move 2:

This move is the same as Move 1 but the right knee is flexed to 90 degrees and moved laterally with the left hand while the therapist makes an oblique move with their right thumb across the the left erector spinae muscle below the lowest rib.

Health Problems that may be assisted

- Any kidney problems

- Nausea

- Fatigue

- Back pain

- Edema

- Incontinence

- Lymphatic drainage

- Scoliosis or pain in the thoracic spine

- Urinary bladder or tract infections

- Migraines or headaches

- Skin problems

Special Comments

Clients often report darker urine after this procedure, which indicates stimulation of the kidneys and release of excess toxic substances. This procedure is one of the lymphatic drainage sequences.

12. Sacral Procedure

This procedure addresses the sacral area of the lower back and takes only a few seconds with often amazing results for relieving pain. It is excellent for pregnant women who commonly suffer back pain as well as being beneficial for pain during menstruation.

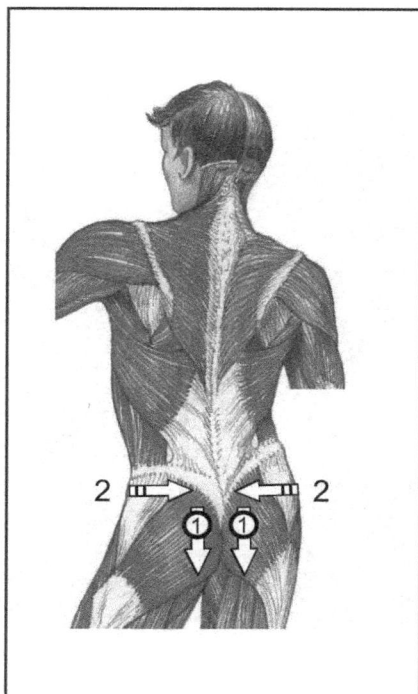

Prerequisite: Moves 1 to 8 of the Lower back procedure

Preparation: The client is in a standing position, bent forward with head lifted up, legs hip- width apart and arms holding the table.

Move 1:

The therapist places their right thumb on the top of the left sacrum approximately 2.5 cm (1 inch) left of the midline of the body. Firm pressure is applied while palpating progressively downwards to the point where only soft tissue is felt. The therapist draws the skin slack upwards (superiorly) and then with firm pressure makes a move downwards (inferiorly). The thumb is then removed for five seconds and then returned to the starting position. This is now a holding point, where firm pressure is applied while Move 2 is applied.

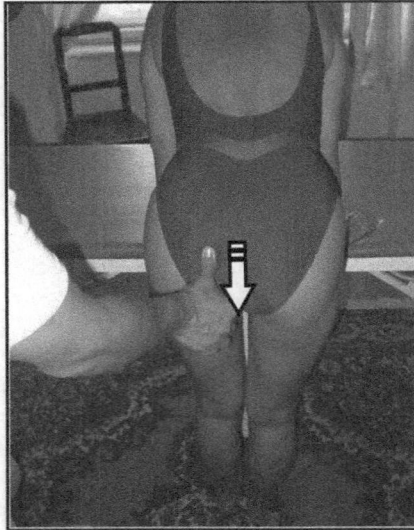

Move 2:

The therapist places their other thumb at the midpoint of the upper border of the **gluteus maximus** muscle. The skin slack is drawn back laterally across the upper border, firm pressure is applied and a medial move is made across the upper border of the gluteus maximus muscle.

Repeat Moves 1 and 2 for the right side of the sacral area of the client.

Health Problems that may be assisted

- During pregnancy to reduce back pain

- Any pain in the sacral area

- Menstrual difficulties

Special Comments:

This procedure is one of the few Bowen procedures that can be performed daily and is especially useful for relief of back pain.

13. Headache Procedure

I often use this procedure at the very end of the Bowen session because it is so effective for calming the nervous system and reducing stress. It is commonly used for any headache pain or migraines and is remarkably effective for cases of anxiety and feelings of nausea.

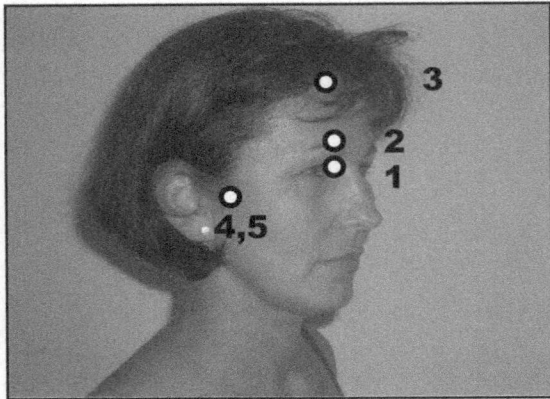

Preparation: The client lies on their back. This procedure involves a series of holding points.

Holding point 1: Both middle fingers are placed on the inner corners of the client's eyes and pressure is applied and held.

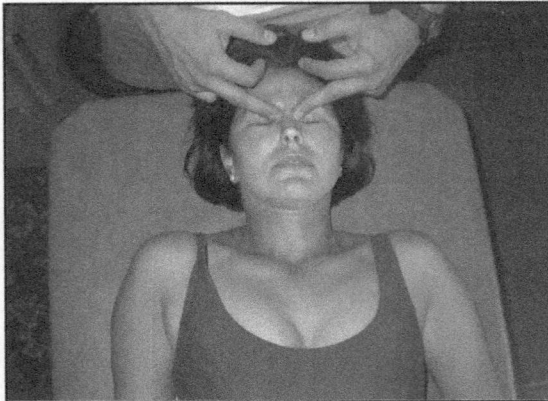

Holding point 2: Holding point 1 is held for two seconds after which both index fingers apply pressure over the eyebrows. This is holding point 2. Holding point 1 is then released.

Holding point 3: Holding point 2 is held for two seconds after which both thumbs apply pressure at the hairline. This is holding point 3. Holding point 2 is then released.

Holding point 4: Holding point 3 is held for two seconds after which both ring fingers apply pressure on the temple. This is holding point 4. Holding point 3 is then released.

Maintain pressure on holding point 4 for two seconds and then return to holding point 1.

Holding points 1 to 4 are repeated four times.

Holding point 5: Apply pressure on holding point 4 with the palms of both hands for approximately 5 to 8 seconds.

Health Problems that may be assisted

- Stress

- Headaches or migraines

- Anxiety

- Nausea

- Dizziness

Special Comments

This is an excellent procedure for reducing stress and for headache pain.

14. Elbow and Wrist Procedure

This procedure addresses elbow and wrist complaints, which commonly include conditions like tennis elbow, carpal tunnel syndrome, sprains, poor circulation or poor nerve innervation.

It can also be used to complement the frozen shoulder procedure in the event of any shoulder problems.

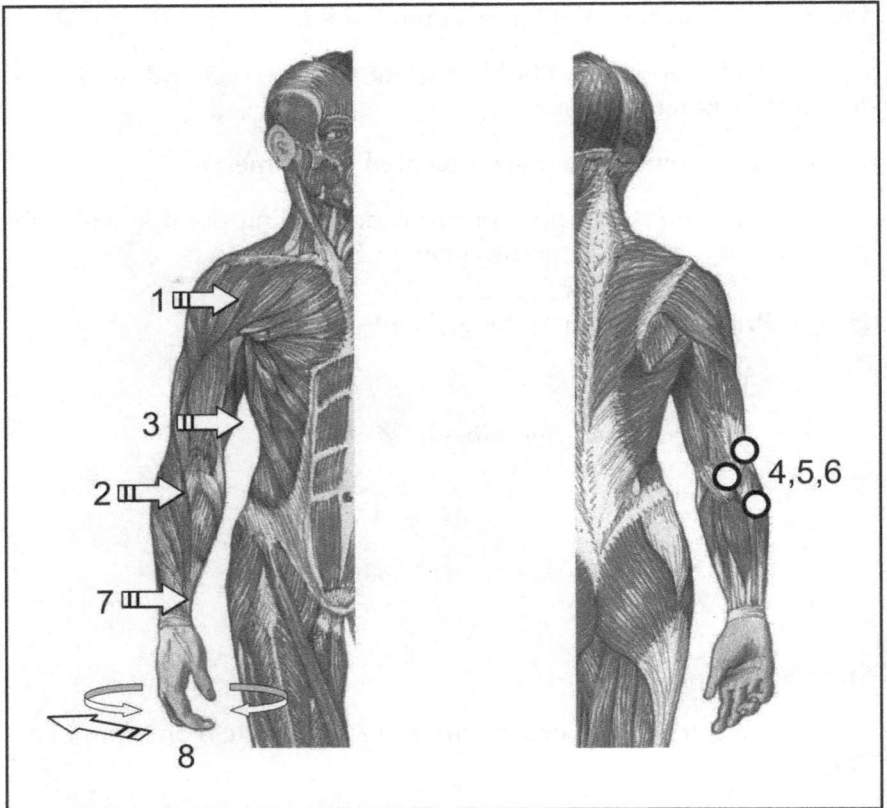

Prerequisite: Moves 1 to 8 of the Upper and mid-back procedure. Turn the client on their back and perform Moves 1 to 6 of the Neck and shoulders procedure

Preparation: The client sits in a chair or on the massage table. The therapist stands on the side of the client.

Move 1:

The therapist places their fingers or thumb on the lateral mid-point of the **deltoid** muscle. The skin slack is drawn back posteriorly and a move is made in the forward (anterior) direction.

Move 2:

The therapist places the thumb of the upper hand on the **extensor digitorum communis** muscle and draws the skin slack back in the ulnar direction and then performs a move in the direction of the radius across the extensor digitorum communis muscle.

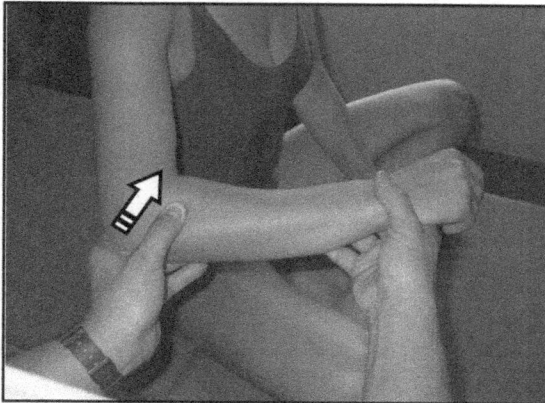

Move 3:

The therapist firmly places their middle finger medially to the **biceps brachii** muscle up from (proximal to) the elbow into the soft tissue where the brachial artery is located. A medial move is then made.

Holding points 4, 5 and 6

The therapist places the tip of the thumb between the humerus and the head of the radius. **This is holding point 4.**

The therapist places the tip of the index finger on the medial aspect of the arm approximately 2 cm (1 inch) posterior to the medial epicondyle. **This is holding point 5.**

The therapist places the tip of the middle finger distal and anterior to the medial epicondyle. **This is holding point 6.**

The therapist firmly applies pressure on all three points for a maximum of ten seconds or until the client feels a tingling sensation in the arms or elbow.

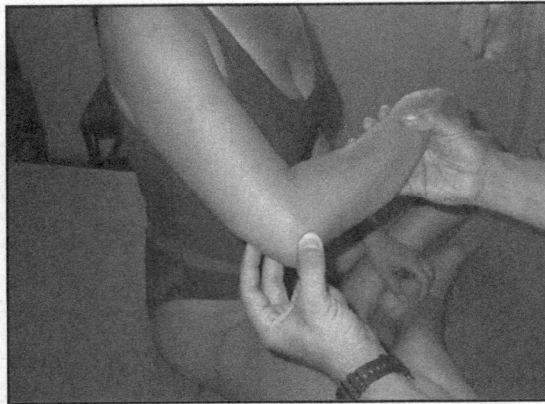

Move 7:

The therapist places their thumb on the midpoint of the client's wrist, on the opposite side of the palm. The skin slack is drawn back in the direction of the ulna and then a move is made with medium pressure in the direction of the radius across the tendons of the **extensor indicis** and **extensor digitorum communis** muscles.

Move 8:

The therapist with both hands performs circumduction of the client's wrists with a number of gentle and incomplete turns with the client's wrist slightly extended. The move is completed by raising the client's upper limb while flexing the wrist and then allowing the relaxed limb to drop down under its own weight, causing extension of the wrist.

The procedure is followed by a special exercise that extends the wrist and arm.

Health Problems that may be assisted

- Any injury or pain in the arm, elbow or hand
- Insufficient circulation to the hands
- Any nerve problems
- Shoulder problems
- Tennis elbow
- Carpel tunnel syndrome

Special Comments

This procedure is one of the most complicated of the Bowen sequences and consists of a series of moves that are performed on the shoulder, elbow and wrist.

A special exercise is performed after the procedure that involves first a slow extension of the wrist and arm followed by a rapid extension. The Bowen therapist must be there to supervise this exercise.

15. Breast Tenderness Procedure

This procedure addresses any kind of pain in the breast such as can occur during premenstrual syndrome, cysts, mastitis as well as problems during lactation. As a lymphatic drainage procedure it is also very effective during flu and fever conditions.

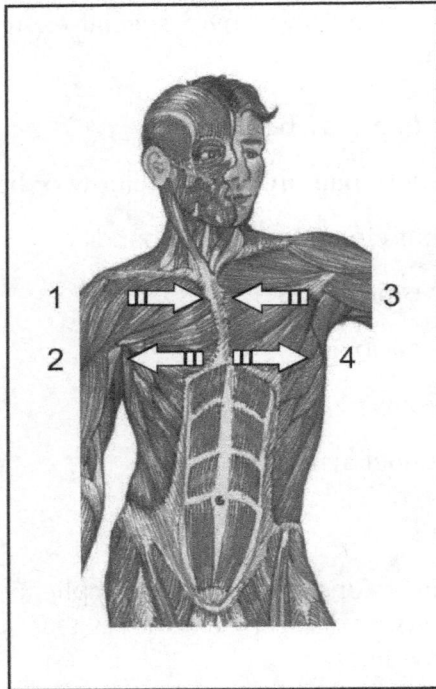

Preparation: The client lies on their back, arms by their side. The therapist stands on the client's left side.

Move 1:

The therapist places both their hands together, palms facing outwards, ulnar border upwards. The radial side of the hand is placed above the opposite breast and the breast tissue is moved slightly downwards (inferiorly). The skin slack is drawn back in the lateral direction and then a medial move is made with firm pressure applied by only the upper hand, over the anterior part of the **pectoralis major** muscle.

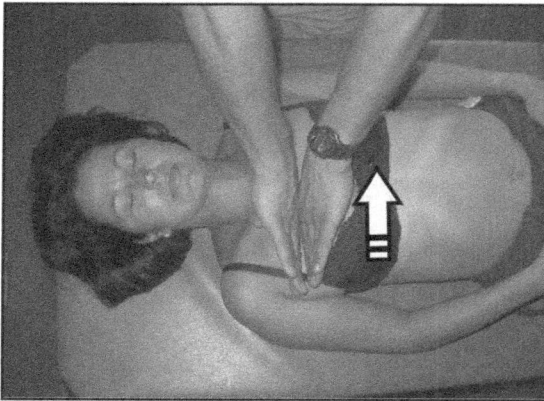

Move 2:

This move is the same as Move 1, except the hands are placed below the opposite breast and the breast tissue is moved slightly upwards (superiorly). The skin slack is drawn back in the medial

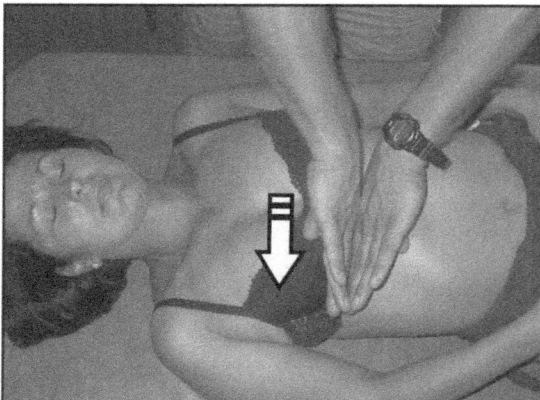

direction and then a lateral move is made across the anterior part of the lower **pectoralis major** and **serratus anterior** muscles.

The therapist stands on the right side of the client.

Move 3:

This move is the same as Move 1, except on the other side of the client.

Move 4:

This move is the same as Move 2, except on the other side of the client.

Health Problems that may be assisted

- Cysts in the breasts
- Breast pain
- Edema
- Fever
- Flu
- Lactation problems or inconsistent milk production
- Lymphatic drainage
- Mastitis
- Pain in the pectoral muscles
- Premenstrual syndrome

Special Comments

This procedure must not be used on women with silicone breast implants.

This procedure is one of the lymphatic drainage sequences.

16. Ankle Procedure

This procedure addresses the ankle and is very effective in cases of swelling or sprains.

It improves circulation to the area allowing for greater healing capacity.

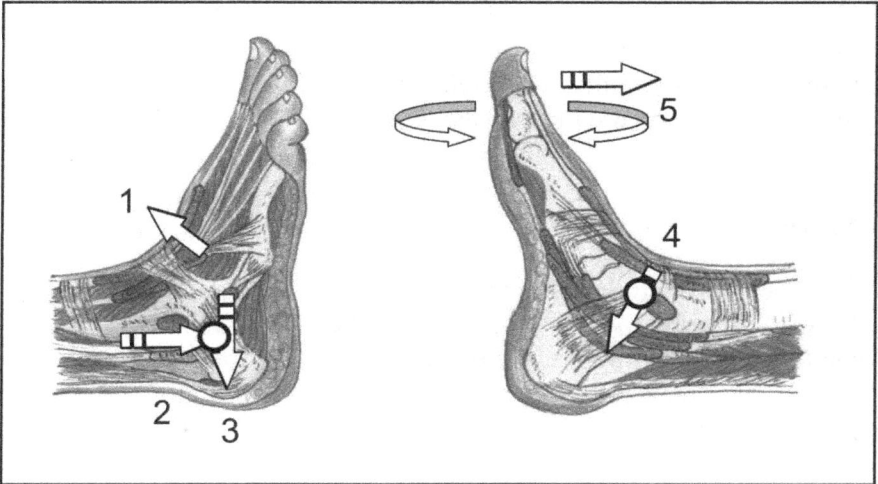

Preparation: Therapist elevates the client's leg and sits on the medial side of the client's ankle.

The moves below are indicated for the left ankle.

Move 1:

The therapist uses their right hand to hold the client's left foot in dorsiflexion. The thumb or finger is placed laterally on the anterior tibial neurovascular bundle. The skin slack is drawn back laterally and then a move is made medially across the tendon of the **extensor hallicis longus**.

Move 2:

The therapist maintains hold of the client's left foot with their right hand and places their left index finger on the lower border of the lateral malleolus. The skin slack is drawn back upwards (superiorly) and then a gentle move is made downwards (inferiorly).

Move 3:

In the ending position of Move 2, the left index finger moves the skin slack back in the medial direction and then a lateral move is made over the calcaneo-fibular ligament. The therapist then releases pressure on the index finger but maintains position until Move 4 is performed.

Move 4:

The therapist places their left thumb below the medial malleolus on the saphenous nerve and vein. The skin slack is drawn back laterally and then a gentle medial move is performed.

Move 5:

The therapist maintains their left index finger and left thumb as holding points as in Move 3 and 4. While holding these points gen-

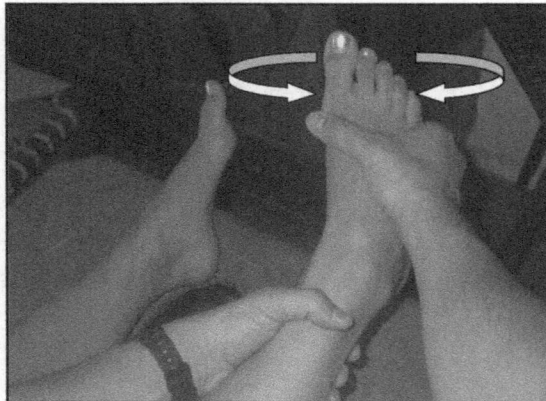

tly, the therapist rotates the client's foot for a few seconds in the clockwise and counter-clockwise directions. Then while applying firm pressure on the holding points and directing force distally, the ankle is thrust into dorsiflexion.

Health Problems that may be assisted

- Any injury or pain in the ankle

- Sprained ankle

- Swelling in the ankle area

Special Comments

The ankle may need to be strapped for support.

For suspected fractures, the client should seek medical attention.

BOWEN THERAPY

Tom Bowen's gift to the world

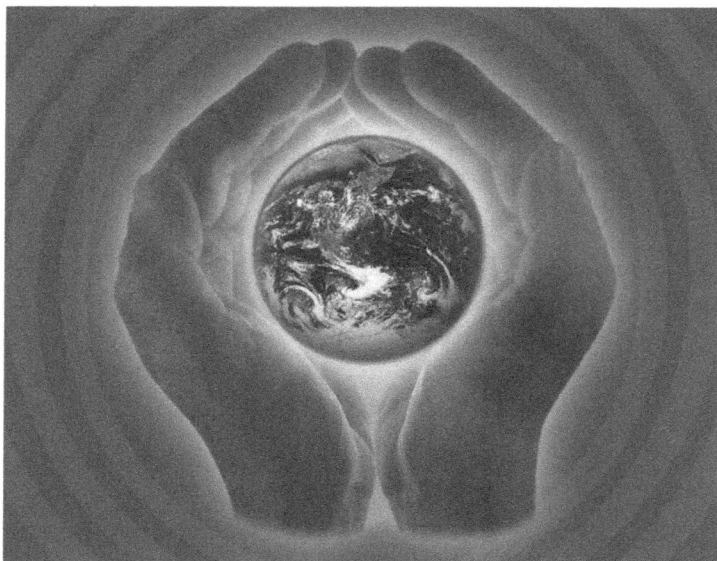

Part 5

After your session

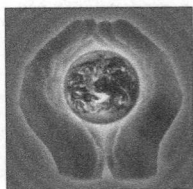

Essential protocol <u>after</u> your Bowen session

14

So, you have just undergone your first Bowen session and are now faced with what to do next. To allow the Bowen method to activate the energy channels in your body and to assist you in promoting a healing environment during your time between Bowen sessions, it is important to follow these important guidelines.

Important protocol on the same day right after your Bowen session:

1. If you feel dizzy after your Bowen session, inform your Bowen therapist, lie down immediately and allow some time for rest until it passes. In most cases, any feelings of instability should pass after a minute or so but allow ten to fifteen minutes to be sure.

2. Do not plan too many activities on the same day after your Bowen session. In many cases, clients feel pleasantly tired and often lightheaded. Avoid exercising or any strenuous activity immediately after your Bowen session. Give your body a chance to rest and to adjust.

3. On the same day of your Bowen session, afterwards do not sit or lie down longer than 30 minutes without spending a few seconds to allow a stretch or short walk. This is required only on the same day of your Bowen session up to bedtime. This protocol allows the body to adapt to the minute changes that can occur in spinal adjustment and promotes lymphatic drainage and toxin removal.

4. Ensure that your body is adequately hydrated, by drinking plenty of water and make sure to avoid heavy fatty meals.

Important protocol after your Bowen session and before your next session:

1. Do not book for your next Bowen session earlier than five days or later than ten days. It is important to allow Bowen to do its work on the body so that muscle tension can be relieved and energy channels can be balanced. An ideal time between sessions is one week.

2. Do not undergo any other body therapy including physiotherapy, reflexology, massage or others during your Bowen sessions and for five days after your last Bowen session. This recommendation serves two purposes. One, it allows your Bowen therapist to monitor the results effectively after each session. The other reason is that any other body therapy may confuse the signals that have been introduced by the Bowen method and reduce its effectiveness.

3. Between your Bowen sessions do not engage in any rigorous exercise. As a general rule reduce any physical activity that you normally engage in to about 60 percent.

4. Drink, Drink, Drink - at least 1.5 liters of fresh, unsweetened, uncarbonated water daily. This is extremely important especially between your Bowen sessions. The Bowen method often results in a release of toxins from the body, which may cause fatigue, nausea and other symptoms especially if not enough water is ingested to allow the body to cleanse. The Bowen method works best under ideal conditions where the body is adequately hydrated and receives a fresh supply of water daily. Remember that drinks and products that contain caffeine such as coffee, black tea, cocoa or chocolate as well as alcohol are diuretics that promote water loss from the body. If you consume any of these products, you will have to increase your water intake even more. As a general rule, for every cup of coffee, add half a liter of water on top of the 1.5 liters that is recommended daily. Drinking water will also reduce the

chance of any negative reactions that may result during the healing process.

5. Try to reduce stress to a minimum if at all possible. Your mind and body should be in as much a relaxed state as possible to allow the body the best chance to heal itself. Avoid conflicting situations that increase stress levels and take time to relax or meditate daily.

6. Do not subject the body to heat or cold after or between your Bowen sessions. This means refraining from hot or cold baths or showers, sauna or steam baths. Try to maintain water at lukewarm temperatures only, to remain closer to your body temperature. Again, the Bowen method has been shown to be more effective under these conditions.

7. Try to avoid crossing your legs when you are in a seated position or any other unnatural movements that can put a strain on your back. Most of these types of movements place tension on one side of the body, which is exactly what the Bowen method is attempting to correct.

8. Ensure that your diet is healthy and that you eat regularly. Remember and ensure adherence to all the holistic factors, including good nutrition and exercise that promote a healing environment.

Following the above recommendations will provide optimum conditions for your body to achieve its goal of attaining a positive healing environment where it has the best chance to heal itself and regain balance or equilibrium. Remember, most of the work that occurs on the body happens after the Bowen session, not during. You may find instant relief of pain in some cases right after your session, but the major regeneration of the body occurs afterwards and depending on the individual, the time that the body needs to heal varies. I believe that the Bowen method should never be used as an instant cure so that you can go on abusing your body and when something hurts return back to the massage table. This is not an intelligent approach to your health. Learn from your mistakes, and listen to your body's messages. The pain you are experiencing is a warning sign, informing you to change your dietary habits or lifestyle. The Bowen method is a technique that rebalances the body so that the healing process is better assisted. After your Bowen session it is up to you to provide the optimum conditions and make improvements in your diet and lifestyle that will allow regeneration of your body. Use Bowen therapy as a catalyst to restart the healing process and motivate yourself to change some of your unhealthy diet and lifestyle habits to ensure a long and healthy life free of pain and chronic health problems.

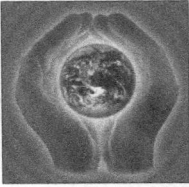

Possible negative reactions and the Healing crisis

This chapter is devoted to possible negative reactions that may occur after Bowen therapy, how to minimize them and what to watch out for. Although the term "negative" is used, I really believe that the unpleasant reactions that sometimes occur after the Bowen method are the body's natural means of dealing with disease and should be looked at as "positive" events during the course of treatment. Over my many years of using the Bowen method I can probably count on one hand the amount of times that I have seen negative reactions where the client had to really stop their sessions. On the other hand, minor negative reactions can occur in my experience up to about 20 percent of the time, so it is important to understand why they occur and what methods can be used to assist or minimize their occurrence.

In order to understand why negative reactions occur in the first place, a short lesson on the Healing Crisis will hopefully help make things more clear.

The Healing Crisis and our return to health

Our body goes through a remarkable sequence of events on the journey to its return to health. As we know, very few individuals are truly healthy and very few that are being treated for medical problems will really become cured. The return to health is not as easy as popping a few pills and waiting until the symptoms go away. The return to health requires all living tissues to regenerate, replacing old cells with new. This requires that organs must pass through a series of stages before they are completely healed. As we start to give our body what it needs to regenerate, our tissues pass through these stages and it is common to experience a Healing Crisis.

What do we mean by the Healing Crisis?

Maybe some of you have noticed that when you begin a new diet or a new cleansing program, some unpleasant side effects occurred. You may have found that changes in the complexion occurred such as acne, boils or skin rashes. I often find that many patients of mine who undergo the Bowen method or begin a vitamin and supplement program along with a change in diet, complain of aches and pains, runny nose, fever, nausea or fatigue. At times it may appear that their condition worsens. It is also common to see that old injuries begin to become more sensitive or begin to hurt when they haven't for many years. Why is this happening, when they are making positive changes or changing their diet and lifestyle for the better? This is what I call the Healing Crisis. Usually it only lasts a few days or weeks but can occur many times on the road to optimum health. I have come to understand that it is a necessary evil that many must go through if they really want to be totally cured and free of disease.

What is really happening during a Healing Crisis?

I believe that when people pass through a healing crisis, their body is trying to rid itself of harmful waste products and acidity in the form of phlegm and discharge. A Healing Crisis is also a time where old injuries, accidents or operations can flare up and become painful as perhaps they may have not been completed healed. Occasionally there is too much of a load on the cleansing organs so feelings of fatigue and sickness occur as well as possible skin problems, indicating the need to rid the body of accumulated waste products. The Bowen method, through its stimulation of the lymphatic system, nervous system and energy channels promotes detoxification of the body but at times it can be too much and negative reactions occur. The problem with most people is that as soon as some of these negative reactions occur, they have a tendency to blame it on the method and often search for another way to cure their health problem. They often run to a doctor for a prescription or a painkiller that only serves to suppress their medical problem and does not promote a healing environment or allow their chronic condition to surface. Symptoms are relieved and the pain is gone but the condition will only come back again and the core or cause of the problem will not be resolved.

Think of a Healing Crisis as a positive event

The body always reacts for a good reason. We cannot fool our bodies with temporary measures as with superficial treatment with drugs, we can only fool ourselves. The Healing Crisis should be viewed as a positive event, not a negative one. Think of it this way, with each healing crisis, the body comes closer to achieving true optimum health and healing. When you start a new health program that may include the Bowen method, exercise or nutritious foods, look forward to a number of healing crises along the way. With each step, the body can eliminate toxins and waste material in a natural drug-free way, those that have often accumulated over many years. Believe in your body. It has amazing regenerative powers that even the greatest minds of today still cannot understand. Believe that with each healthy lifestyle change you make, the body will respond in a natural way and begin to regenerate tissues and organs that may have been ignored for many years. In order for the body to accomplish this it often comes with a small price. You may feel that your condition is getting worse at times but if you persevere and make it through the many healing crises that you encounter, I truly believe that you will find the road to achieving the optimum health that you deserve.

What are some negative reactions that may occur as a result of undergoing the Bowen method?

Do not be surprised if you experience any of these reactions for a short time after you have undergone the Bowen method. Usually they pass after a few days and with time become minimal.

Headaches

Pain or sensitivity in the area of old injuries, scars or operations.

Fever

Nausea

Dizziness

Anxiety

Nervousness

Back pain

Swollen glands

Skin irritations

Acne

Boils

Extreme fatigue

Stiffness in muscles or joints

Flu-like symptoms

Edema

Increased frequency of urination

Constipation or diarrhea

How can these negative reactions be minimized?

Probably the most important recommendation to minimize the healing crisis is to drink plenty of clean, fresh water. This will provide a medium for waste products to flush the body rather than allowing them to stay in, which can lead to headaches, fatigue, fever, swollen glands and other symptoms. Follow the essential protocol that was discussed in the previous chapter and ensure regular exercise in moderation. Do not make too many diet and lifestyle changes at once, make them gradually step-by-step. This will allow the body to adapt and will minimize the chance of an overload of toxins all at once, which can be too much for you to handle.

Welcome your healing crisis. Do not suppress the body's natural processes by anti-cold remedies, anti-inflammatory, anti-allergy medicines or pain medications. They only serve to slow down the body's attempts to heal itself. The more we have suppressed our medical problems over our lifetime, the greater the occurrence of healing crisis as we begin to self-heal. I understand that in some cases extreme back pain or migraines are so debilitating that it is hard to live without any pain medication. Try to use it only if necessary and search for natural healing products if at all possible.

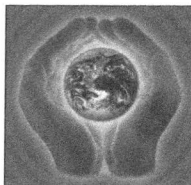

When Bowen does not work as well as expected

It would be dishonest to say that Bowen therapy works for everyone, every time. Such a method unfortunately does not exist in the world today. I have seen patients of mine who have responded favorably to the Bowen method yet acupuncture or other methods did not work for them and vice versa. Remember, we are all different and we respond in different ways. What I can honestly say is that I have seen significant improvements in over 80 percent of my patients, often after only three Bowen sessions. I believe therefore with such a high success rate, this method yields outstanding results. I have listed some possible reasons why the Bowen method may not have resulted in the success that you expected.

Reasons why your Bowen therapy sessions may have not resulted in success:

Failure to drink enough water during the week

This is often the greatest culprit and major reason why Bowen is often not successful. Failing to drink enough water (minimum 1.5 liters) will slow down the body's ability to self-heal. We cannot expect to achieve a healing environment if our body is denied this life-giving nutrient. Increase this amount if you drink coffee or alcohol beverages.

Taking hot baths or showers

As I have mentioned before, it is recommended that you use only luke-warm water when you bathe or shower. Extreme heat or cold to the area has been found to interfere with the healing process initiated by the Bowen method. For the best results, your body temperature needs to be maintained at normal levels. During your sessions, stay away from saunas, steam baths or hot tubs.

Rigorous exercise

Although it is recommended to engage in moderate exercise between your Bowen sessions, it is not recommended to exercise in excess. This means that if you are an athlete or serious fitness enthusiast, allow your body to rest and reduce your normal work load to 60 percent of what you would usually do.

Not enough sleep

Sleep is a time when our bodies and mind regenerate. You cannot expect positive results from Bowen therapy if you do not have regular and quality sleep.

Poor nutrition

Our bodies are dependent on what we ingest. Our life processes, which include digestion, absorption, circulation, utilization and detoxification, require nutritious foods to maintain their effectiveness. The Bowen method will initiate and stimulate these processes but they have to be supported with quality nutrition in order for regeneration of tissue to occur.

Excess alcohol or caffeine

Other than its known negative effects on the human body, alcohol and caffeine are also strong diuretics that promote water loss. A state of dehydration does not promote a healing environment. The Bowen method as a result will often not yield the outcome you desire.

Too much stress

As we know, stress affects all our body processes. It creates a block for healing and regeneration can be slowed down considerably. The Bowen method is excellent for reducing stress and muscle tension but additional emotional stress between your sessions will not assist in the healing process. Emotional conflicts, arguments, excessive workload in the workplace or personal life will not allow the Bowen method to perform as well as it should.

The problem may require more Bowen sessions

It is possible that more Bowen sessions are required for your chronic health problem. I have seen in some cases that positive results only came after more than three sessions and up to ten sessions.

Poor posture or unnatural movement of the body

Improper posture when seated, poor mattresses when sleeping or any unnatural twisting or turning of the body (includes crossing the legs) can interfere with the Bowen method.

Undergoing other body therapies at the same time

Engaging in other body therapies at the same time as you are undergoing Bowen may confuse the signals in the body, thus negating the positive effects of Bowen therapy.

Drugs or medications

There is such a vast array of drugs on the market today. Some have side effects and others can suppress the healing crisis and slow down regeneration of body tissues. Many have negative effects on detoxification organs such as the liver and as we have learned, detoxification is one of the primary requirements of the body to allow it to self-heal.

The client does not want to be healed

If you do not have the will to live or do not believe in the healing ability of the Bowen method, this will interfere in its success. The power of the will is much stronger than we can imagine.

The Bowen method may not be for you

Again, as I mentioned not every healing method is for everyone. You may be one of the few who will achieve better results if you try another method other than Bowen. Before you come to this conclusion however, ensure that you have followed all the recommendations in this book and have given the best possible chance for Bowen to do its work.

I can truly say that in my long-time practice using Bowen therapy on thousands of patients, I have come across only very few for whom it would not be beneficial. In most cases one or more of the above recommendations were not being adhered to and the client did not achieve the best that Bowen could offer. Bowen therapy is exactly what I have stated a few times already in this book, a catalyst that initiates the healing process, but we must be prepared to do some work on improving our diet and lifestyle habits to completely rid ourselves of the health problems or back pain that we suffer from.

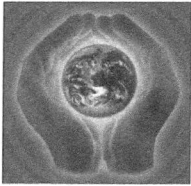

Bowen therapy, relieving stress and psychological reactions

One of the many reasons why clients choose to undergo Bowen therapy is because of negative feelings due to the build-up of stress. This problem is becoming more and more common in today's hectic world. Life often becomes very impersonal and the human need for touch is ignored leading to increases in stress levels and psychological problems. It is no wonder that more and more people find psychological relief and can cope much better after Bowen therapy. Before we discuss some of the amazing reactions to the Bowen method, let's take a look at the meaning of stress and what it can do to the body.

What is Stress?

Stress occurs when our bodies experience "wear and tear" as we adjust to the environment around us that is continually changing. It is a factor that has both a physical and emotional effect on us and can result in positive or negative feelings. On the positive side, stress influences us to take action and to become more aware of our environment. On the negative side, it can result in feelings of anxiety, distrust, anger or depression, which in turn can lead to health problems such as headaches, upset stomach, insomnia, ulcers, backaches, high blood pressure, heart disease, cancer or stroke. With every life change such as the birth of a child, move to another city or country, job promotion, marriage, divorce or death of a loved one, we experience stress as we readjust our lives. Throughout this period of adjustment, stress will either assist us or hinder us depending on how we react to it.

What does stress do to the body?

Although this is a very difficult question and still an issue that is currently being studied, we do know that some people handle stress better than others. When there is excess stress, for some people, it can make them feel like they are not in control of their lives. When stress builds up the heart beats faster, and digestion, circulation, as well as all the essential life processes are drastically affected. When they are not functioning optimally it is no surprise that it can result in damage to the body. Stress has been linked to very serious diseases such as cancer, heart problems, high blood pressure and stroke. Stress can lead to so many different symptoms from tightening of the muscles and headaches to disruption of menstrual cycles and back pain.

How can the Bowen method assist in reducing stress?

Remember back at the beginning of this book, when I discussed balance and homeostasis? Without balance, our bodily functions and psychological state are in chaos and it becomes difficult for the body to function smoothly. In this kind of state, toxins and free radicals accumulate in the body and feelings of anxiety, stress, aggression or depression are common. An unhealthy and unbalanced body influences greatly our psychological behavior and makes it difficult to adjust to the changing environment around us. Hence, we begin to feel the effects of stress.

The Bowen method, by rebalancing the functions of the body and stimulating the nervous, muscular, circulatory and detoxification systems, allows the body to regain homeostasis so that regeneration of body tissues becomes much easier. As the body becomes better able to rid itself of harmful toxins and muscle tension is released, stress is reduced. It seems that Bowen therapy has much more benefits than just the physical.

What are possible psychological reactions?

Although the Bowen method is not used intentionally to evoke psychological reactions it is very common to encounter them in practice. Often deeply suppressed emotions can surface after release of muscle tension in the body. Do not be surprised if you feel like crying or if you experience any kind of emotional outbursts. Your mind and body are communicating and reminding you that they must work together in balance to provide the quality health that you require. As we learned earlier about the healing crisis, a healing environment requires that all physical and emotional health problems reach the surface.

There are just so many psychological reactions that have been reported by my patients but I have included some of the most common ones below:

Emotional release

An emotional release can come as an overwhelming feeling for many people and can range from extreme happiness, sudden fatigue, mood change or crying. It can occur during a Bowen session or days afterwards.

Feelings of euphoria

I have witnessed many people who report feelings of euphoria or extreme happiness and they often report feeling as if they were a little intoxicated.

Increased energy levels

In some cases especially right after Bowen therapy, people may feel high energy levels and may report difficulty in sleeping that night.

Feelings of lightness or a heavy load being taken off

These feelings of lightness are commonly reported along with euphoria and as stress is released, clients may compare it to a load being lifted off the body.

Deep suppressed feelings come to the surface

Even during Bowen therapy, clients can achieve a state of relaxation and comfort, which will allow suppressed feelings to come to the surface. For some clients this means that they will talk more about emotional problems that they may have experienced or that they experience outbreaks of crying or intense emotional release. This is a very positive event and can result in dramatic health improvements.

Relief from negative emotions

An unhealthy mind and body that is full of toxins often reduces energy levels and results in pre-occupation with negative feelings such as grief, distrust, anger, hatred, revenge or jealousy. As a result of the Bowen method, negative feelings are often reduced, people start to think more clearly and adopt a more positive outlook on life.

Feelings of calmness

The body, mind and spirit need to be in balance to achieve harmony. With harmony comes a feeling of calmness and control. I think everyone has a desire to achieve a sense of calm and many Bowen patients report feelings like this after their sessions.

Feelings of better concentration and focus

The world is full of distractions and information that often cause us to lose focus on what is really important. It is common to encounter feelings of anxiety and to lose concentration. Bowen patients often report that they can focus or concentrate on tasks much better.

Improvement in anxiety

A build-up of stress can lead to anxiety attacks where you can lose control over your life. I have witnessed countless cases where cases of anxiety were dramatically improved.

Improvements in creative energy

I have had writers who suffered from writer's block where the Bowen method has assisted as well as many cases where clients reported improvements in creative energy, formation of ideas and problem solving.

Feelings of being more alert and increased awareness

In some cases, patients feel pleasant fatigue after Bowen therapy but in other cases clients have reported the opposite. These people have reported that they feel more alert and aware of what is happening around them.

Feelings of reassurance, increased confidence and being more in control

Many clients feel a greater sense of safety and reassurance. As they gain more control over their health, they often report feelings of greater self-confidence. I have personally witnessed this occurring with application of the Bowen method, especially with cases of women with eating disorders such as bulimia or anorexia or victims of sexual abuse.

Feelings of being understood

Many people can feel lost or misguided and their health problems can be a confusing experience. They may even feel that not even their doctor or loved ones can understand their problems. Many clients after Bowen therapy have reported that they feel a better sense of being understood.

Outbursts of crying or laughing

Outbursts of crying are most common in women but I have witnessed them even in men. I have seen people have laughing fits, or become extremely over-emotional. Just like a sad movie or intense physical trauma has the ability to cause us to cry, Bowen therapy's relaxing effect on the mind and body often has similar effects. As suppressed emotions surface within the healing environment that is assisted by the Bowen method, these outbursts can occur and are a sign that the mind and body are communicating and rebalancing.

BOWEN THERAPY

Tom Bowen's gift to the world

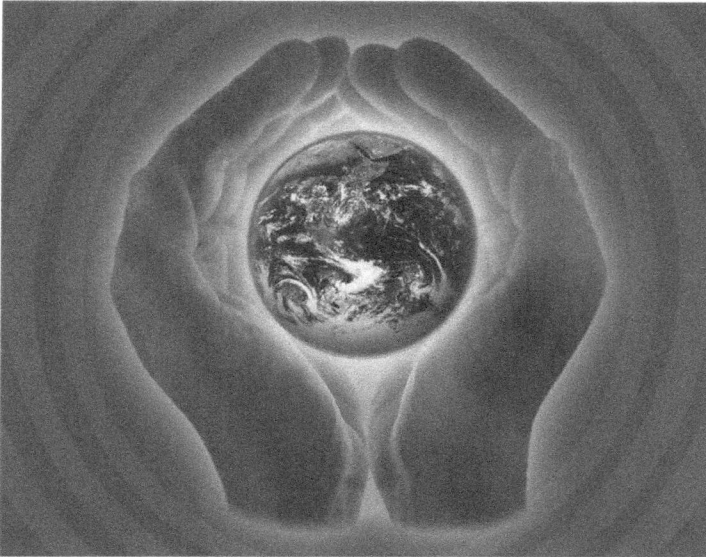

Part 6

Case studies, special thoughts and patient comments

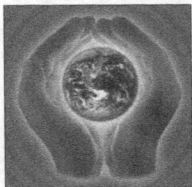

Case studies from the naturopathic practice of Frank Navratil, BSc. N.D. 18

Over the many years that I have used Bowen therapy in practice, I have come across just so many success stories, not in every case but over 80 percent of them had positive results. I have included just a small sample of some of the most remarkable cases that I have personally witnessed. They serve as examples of how powerful and effective Bowen therapy can be and how in many cases this method has the amazing ability to reactivate the body's capability to heal itself.

1. LOWER BACK PAIN Woman 46 years old

Client History: This woman had chronic lower back pain for ten years, found it very difficult to bend over, visited several specialists over the years and had tried acupuncture and many other methods with no significant relief. When I met her she was taking several pain- relief medications, she was barely able to climb a set of stairs and doctors recommended surgery. Due to her illness she was unable to work.

Results after Bowen Therapy: After only the first Bowen session, all back pain disappeared the following day. Two days later it returned and lasted for two days, after which all pain disappeared and she was able to completely stop taking all pain medications. When I saw her after a week for her second session, she was ecstatic; her mood had changed from deep depression to positive and hopeful. She came again for the third time after a week and told me that the pain did not come back all week, she was able to bend over without any pain and she threw away all her medications. She called me a month later just to thank me for changing her whole life, as the pain had stayed away for a whole month for the first time in ten years. She was now even able to exercise.

2. MIGRAINE HEADACHES Woman 32 years old

Client History: This young woman had undergone a fair amount of stress and gone through a divorce in the past. She had suffered migraine headaches for several years that were so debilitating that she would have to take time off work. The frequency of these migraines was three or four times a month and would often last for a day or more. The only relief she could find was through medications that her doctor had prescribed.

Results after Bowen Therapy: After the first Bowen session, the day after she reported feeling light-headed, but full of energy. The next day her migraine came back even worse than before and she called me in a panic and I convinced her to be patient, to drink plenty of water and eat regular healthy meals. Her migraine subsided in two days and when she returned for her second session she was pain-free but afraid that the Bowen session would trigger another attack. Nevertheless after some convincing, she decided to try again. Her migraine this time did not come back and when she came for number three, she had a much more positive attitude. I did not hear from her until after six months. When she called me she told me for the first time in several years she had not had one migraine headache for six months, which she found almost impossible to believe. After six months, she experienced a migraine but it was much less intense than they had been previously but she booked in again for another three sessions with me. I did not hear back from her again.

3. URINARY TRACT INFECTION Woman 25 years old

Client History: This client suffered from chronic urinary tract infections several times a year. When she arrived she was suffering from intense burning pain.

Results after Bowen Therapy: Right after the first Bowen session was over, the burning pain completely subsided. She came back again after a few months with another urinary tract infection and the procedure was repeated again with the same success. She was advised to increase her fluid intake, abstain from coffee, sweets and white flour products. I performed Bowen another two times to assist in promoting kidney function and toxin removal. Her urinary tract infections did not come back this time.

4. CHRONIC CONSTIPATION Male 55 years old

Client History: This man had suffered many years from chronic constipation and could only have one bowel movement a week and only with the help of chemical laxatives. He was experiencing extreme fatigue and suffering from hemorrhoids.

Results after Bowen Therapy: Half way through his first Bowen session, he began to experience an unusual feeling in his stomach and digestive tract. He told me that he had to go to the toilet. He informed that the procedure had caused him to have a bowel movement. I told him that this could occur initially but that he would have to put some work into it, including increasing water and fiber intake and exercise. He reported feeling euphoria after the session and full of energy. He came back for his second session and could hardly wait to tell me that he had a bowel movement every day since his first session and without one laxative. On the third session, he looked and felt much better, and reported having sometimes two bowel movements a day.

5. ASTHMA Woman 52 years old

Client History: This woman had suffered from asthma for at least 15 years. She would regularly have to use a bronchial dilator spray and often had several attacks every month.

Results after Bowen Therapy: After the first session, she complained that coughing increased and she began to cough up phlegm. This subsided after a few days and when she arrived for her second session, she reported improvement in breathing capacity, describing it like a "weight lifted off the chest." I performed four more Bowen sessions over the following few weeks with gradual improvements every week. She was eventually able to stop using her bronchial dilator spray, her breathing cleared and energy levels dramatically improved.

6. EMOTIONAL RELEASE Male 35 years old

Client History: This man was a physiotherapist and just told me that he was under a lot of stress at the moment. He was quiet and seemed a bit introverted.

Results after Bowen Therapy: This was an unusual case although I had seen this kind of reaction many times in women but never in a man. Half way through the procedure, he asked me to stop and informed me that he was feeling very strange. He started to shake and tremble uncontrollably and I asked him to lie down for a few minutes until it passes. Eventually he began to cry and could no longer hold back the tears. He continued to tremble and cry in this state for a few minutes after which he calmed down, felt very embarrassed and immediately became extremely tired. He slept on the massage table for a half hour before he woke. I thought it might be better to stop at that moment, explained to him that he just went through an emotional release and he agreed to book in for the next session. After a week he came and told me that he almost did not come, as he was still embarrassed about his behavior on the first session but all week he felt so well and was convinced that the Bowen method really works. He felt an incredible weight off his shoulders that he hadn't felt for years. He came for another couple sessions, with no unusual reactions this time but he reported feeling less anxiety, more energy and began to communicate more freely.

7. HIGH BLOOD PRESSURE Man 59 years old

Client History: This patient had suffered from high blood pressure for several years and was taking medications to keep it down. Without medication his blood pressure was 210/100. He was overweight and a past smoker who had quit a year before I saw him.

Results after Bowen Therapy: Before his first Bowen session I took this man's blood pressure and it measured 190/95. After the procedure, only a half hour later, I measured his blood pressure again and it had dropped to 140/90. He reported feeling less pressure in his head and much calmer. Since then I have had a number of high blood pressure patients and have conducted the same test with very similar results. I have also tested pulse rate before and after with similar decreases. Over the next few weeks he came for a few more times, he changed his diet drastically, increased water intake and reduced salt and was able after a few months to reduce his medication and his blood pressure steadily decreased.

8. IMMUNITY Child 14 years old

Client History: He came in with his mother and she informed me that her son was diagnosed with a constant high fever that just would not go away as well as low immune function which resulted in several bouts of flu every year, ear and throat infections. He had been forced to take antibiotics several times a year and his stomach and digestion was suffering as a result.

Results after Bowen Therapy: It took three sessions before any results were achieved. After the third session, the fever went down. After the first session he reported drainage from his nose and ears and an increase in coughing spells. His mother called almost a year later with the news that for the first time in a long time he went throughout the year with not one bout of flu or ear and throat infection. They booked in again for another few sessions for prevention.

9. KNEE INJURY Man 26 years old athlete runner

Client History: This young man was a long distance runner who had injured his knee several times but this time his doctor had recommended surgery and he was set for a knee operation in a couple months. His knee was very swollen and painful. Besides this his health was very good.

Results after Bowen Therapy: After the first Bowen session, he reported warmth around his knee and lower leg. In two days the swelling went down at least fifty percent and when he came back for his second session the swelling and pain was almost gone. He said that he was feeling much better, was experiencing no pain and asked if he could train again. I told him to wait and only go for light brisk walks. After a few more weeks of Bowen sessions he informed me that he had returned back to his doctor feeling almost back to normal and received the good news that an operation was not necessary anymore.

10. TINNITUS Male 65 years old

Client History: This man was experiencing ringing in the ears or tinnitus almost constantly day and night. He said that it was driving his crazy and the only was he could sleep was to keep the radio on so it could distract him from the ringing. He had tried medications and had visited several doctors with no success.

Results after Bowen Therapy: After this man came for his first session he reported that much to his surprise the ringing had increased after his Bowen session and he called to cancel his next appointment. I convinced him that such a reaction is common and that he should still try to come. After much hesitation he agreed, and after his second session the ringing stopped the following day. It came back again after a couple of days but the ringing was now less intense. He tried not taking his medication and was much more positive when he came for his third session. Over the next couple months we worked on it and the ringing gradually decreased until it was only slightly heard and on some days he reported it completely disappeared.

11. ECZEMA Female 22 years old

Client History: This young lady had suffered from recurrent outbreaks of eczema on the elbows and behind the knees. She had poor dietary habits and often complained of constipation.

Results after Bowen Therapy: After the first Bowen session, this client reported that itching had increased in the affected areas. After the second session it stopped. After a few more sessions the eczema completed cleared up. It returned only slightly after six months and she booked in for another few sessions, improved her diet and has not had any problems since.

12. INFERTILITY Female 29 years old

Client History: This client had been taking birth control pills for many years but had stopped and was now trying to have a child with no success for over two years. Her doctor told her that her and her husband were in good condition and there was no reason that she could not have a child.

Results after Bowen Therapy: She came in for three Bowen sessions and reported feeling great each time she returned. After the first session, she had a small emotional release and could not hold back the tears. She later commented how calm and relaxed the Bowen method made her feel. Two months after her last session she called me to thanks me and tell me that she was finally pregnant.

13. LUMP IN THE BREAST Female 44 years old

Client History: This female reported that she suffered from fatigue as well as from lymphatic congestion in the form of edema, swelling in the legs and hands. She had been diagnosed with a liver problem a year before. A lump in her breast was found and she decided to deal with it by coming in for Bowen therapy.

Results after Bowen Therapy: A week after the first Bowen session, the lump disappeared. She was amazed when she came in and also reported less swelling in her legs and hands. After another two sessions, not only was her lump in her breast gone but she felt much more energetic.

14. KIDNEY PROBLEM Female 30 years old

Client History: This woman came in because she had heard that the Bowen method can assist the kidneys. She had bags under her eyes and would suffer from dull pain in the lower back. She suffered from migraines and recurrent skin problems. Most of all she felt tired all the time.

Results after Bowen Therapy: The next day after her first Bowen session she reported that her urine was much darker than usual and this lasted for three days. One week after her second session, she felt so tired that she had to book off work. She called me and I told her that she was probably releasing a lot of toxins from the body and going through a healing crisis and that she should try to be patient and let the body do its work. After the third session, she found that her skin had cleared and she did not feel as tired any more. The dull pain in her lower back area stopped.

15. FROZEN SHOULDER Male 51 years old

Client History: This client came in with a frozen shoulder and he could not lift his arm higher than his shoulder. Any movement of the arm would cause intense pain. He was suffering with this problem for over six months. He was taking pain medication, tried physiotherapy but had no success.

Results after Bowen Therapy: Immediately after the first Bowen session the client was able to lift his arm straight up without feeling any pain. He was amazed. During the week he reported improvements in the range of motion around the shoulder with only occasional pain. After a few weeks he felt completely healed. He told me that doctors and physiotherapists had tried with no success for six months but Bowen therapy had completely treated his problem in just a few weeks.

16. PREMENSTRUAL SYNDROME Female 24 years old

Client History: This lady complained of irregular periods, intense cramping, headaches and tenderness in the breasts every month. She would always have to take painkillers and was forced to frequently take time off of work because of this problem.

Results after Bowen Therapy: She came in during the time of the month where she was experiencing these symptoms and found that the Bowen method completely alleviated all cramping, tenderness and headaches. She came in for a few more sessions and the following month had absolutely no symptoms before her period.

17. DIGESTIVE PROBLEMS Male 46 years old

Client History: This man was having a very difficult time digesting any food. He had worked with me on his diet but still almost anything he ate would cause him pain and discomfort. He would suffer bouts of constipation and then diarrhea. His energy levels were falling and he was afraid that he might be seriously ill.

Results after Bowen Therapy: After three sessions of Bowen therapy his digestive upsets were completely relieved. He was able to eat most foods without suffering pain or discomfort. He found also that symptoms of constipation and diarrhea had also disappeared. As a result he was able to digest more foods and energy levels returned.

18. SEXUAL ABUSE Female 18 years old

Client History: This girl was under extreme stress when I met her for the first time and it was obvious that it was negatively affecting her health. She was suffering from frequent urinary tract infections and had pain from the ovaries.

Results after Bowen Therapy: I performed the first three Bowen sessions and she reported feeling better and the pain had stopped. On the fourth session she had an emotional release and began to cry uncontrollably. She explained that her father had sexually abused her when she was young and only now was trying to work through it. She told me that she had not told anyone about it before. I told her that it was a good sign that she was now talking about it and that she should probably seek counseling. She agreed and continued her Bowen sessions for several weeks. The pain and urinary tract infections did not return. She called me several months later and told me that she was making a lot of progress and thanked me for my help. She was grateful that the Bowen method had assisted her in relieving her psychological pain that she was burdened with for so many years.

19. NECK PAIN Male 33 years old

Client History: This client came to me with extreme neck pain and was not able to turn his head from side to side. He worked a lot at the computer, did not exercise very much and was feeling very tired most days. He admitted that he worked long hours and that his job did not leave him much time for anything else.

Results after Bowen Therapy: After the first Bowen session, he was able to turn to head from side to side with only minimum pain. He came for a couple more sessions and the neck pain completely subsided. I recommended that he start exercising and ensure adequate sleep. He did not require any more treatment.

20. DEPRESSION Female 48 years old

Client History: This lady suffered often from depression and one of her friends had suggested she try the Bowen method as it had helped her in the past. She had been prescribed anti-depressive medication and was very skeptical that the Bowen method would help her at all.

Results after Bowen Therapy: After two Bowen sessions she reported that she felt less anxiety and was able to reduce her medication. After 8 or 9 sessions she found that she experienced depression less often and was convinced that the Bowen method had helped her. I recommended after 10 sessions for her to take a break for a couple months and then resume the Bowen method. She called me after a couple months to say that she had no episodes of depression during the two months and felt that she did not need further treatment.

21. UNEVEN LEG LENGTH Female 28 years old

Client History: This woman was experiencing back and neck pain with frequent headaches. She attributed this to the fact that one leg was longer than the other and she was forced to wear a pad in her shoe to compensate for the difference.

Results after Bowen Therapy: After 4 sessions of the Bowen method all of her back and neck pain subsided and she reported no headaches at all. After the second session, I measured her leg length and there was no discrepancy at all. It seemed that it was the fact that one side of her hip was uneven causing the discrepancy in leg length. The Bowen method released the muscle tension on one side of the body that was causing her pain and at the same time was able to bring the leg back to normal length. She was now able to get rid of the pad that she wore in her shoes.

22. JAW NOISE Male 36 years old

Client History: This man's primary complaint was that whenever he ate or chewed he would hear a clicking sound in his jaw.

Results after Bowen Therapy: After only one session, the clicking noises completely stopped. He came in for two more sessions and the clicking noises never returned.

23. NUMBNESS IN THE HANDS AND LEGS Female 52 years old

Client History: This client complained of numbness in one leg and one arm with prickly sensations. She had a history of back problems due to a car accident that she had many years ago.

Results after Bowen Therapy: After two sessions of the Bowen method, she reported feeling less numbness in her leg and arm. Her back pain that she suffered from was completely relieved after just a few sessions more. After seven sessions, the numbness disappeared.

24. BACK PAIN WITH SHOOTING PAINS IN THE LEGS Female 58 years old

Client History: This woman came to me with extreme lower back pain with shooting pains to the legs. She was significantly overweight and suffering from constipation and gallstones. She was taking painkillers to make it through the week.

Results after Bowen Therapy: One week after her first session, she came and told me that the back pain and shooting pains had completed subsided and she had not felt so good in so many years. I performed a couple more sessions so that the Bowen method could further assist regeneration in her body. After that, her back pain was completely alleviated and she did not need any further treatment. She stopped taking painkillers.

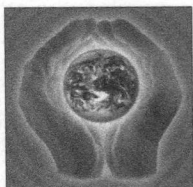

Special thoughts and conditions

I hope that as we approach the end of this book, you have grown to realize how universal the Bowen method is and how it can be applied to people of all ages and with all types of health problems. I also hope that you have also gained some valuable advice on how you can assist your body to heal itself. This chapter summarizes some of the important concepts surrounding Bowen therapy and introduces new applications for some special conditions.

Special thoughts:

1. Treat the person not the disease

One of the most basic principles of holistic medicine is to treat the whole person not just the disease. This is often where modern medicine falls short and often only symptoms are treated but not the cause. The Bowen method follows this important holistic principle. For example, if there is a pain or a problem in a certain area of the body, that area is not the only one where the Bowen method is applied. Other Bowen procedures are prerequisites or used in combination to stimulate the circulation, nervous system and lymphatic system of the whole body. In this way a healing environment is achieved so that the body can better heal itself. Often patients will ask me to spend more time on the area that hurts and I have to reply and explain that the cause of their complaint may be somewhere else so it is important to treat the body as a whole. You can be assured that your whole body will benefit as a result of the Bowen method.

2.   Believe that the body can heal itself

Many patients have been surprised to discover that they
actually have control over their own health. After years
and years of being dependant on their doctors, many eventually come to the conclusion that chemical drugs are only
a superficial means of dealing with chronic disease. Another important principle of Bowen therapy is that it is not
the Bowen procedures that heal the health problem, but
the body that does the work. Given the right conditions,
adequate nutrition and other holistic needs, the body can
heal itself. Bowen therapy is just the catalyst to achieve a
healing environment where tissue can once again regenerate.

3.   Bowen therapy should be only part of the pie of holistic health care for the client

As you have learned, holistic health is composed of many
factors and the Bowen method is only a part of the pie of
holistic health care. In order to be most effective, a healing program should include along with the Bowen method, good nutrition, adequate water intake, regular exercise, clean air as well as all the holistic factors that I discussed back in Chapter 3. If you really want to get to the
core of your health problem and cure it for good, you need
to satisfy all of your holistic needs.

4.   You cannot rush the body's healing processes

As much as we would like to believe, the body's healing
processes cannot be rushed. Each one of us has different
capabilities to self-heal. Do not expect overnight results
and be prepared to put some work into it to become well.
Depending on how much abuse you have subjected your
body to in the past, will determine how much extra work
you need to do to dig yourself out of those chronic health
problems. Try to avoid drugs such as painkillers or anti-
inflammatory medication, if at all possible and let nature

take its course. Expect that you will encounter a healing crisis along the way to your return to health. Bowen therapy can greatly assist in the healing process but can only follow nature's course providing that conditions are favorable in the body to allow regeneration.

5. Create an optimum healing environment

In order for our body to self-heal, an optimum healing environment must be created.

As we have learned earlier, a healing environment often leads to faster recovery from diseases and infection as well as reduction of pain. In order for Bowen therapy to have the best effect, follow the advice on holistic health and give your body the greatest chance to heal itself.

6. Health is influenced by more than just the physical

If you are under a lot of stress or if you are suffering from any psychological problems or depression, this may be contributing to your physical health problems. Examine your lifestyle and your relationships and work on bringing any negative suppressed feelings like hatred, jealousy, resentment or anger to the surface. Bowen therapy, through its activation of energy channels throughout the body assists not only physical health problems but often many psychological problems as well as they begin to surface when the mind and body begin to relax.

7. Treat the cause not just the symptoms

Finally, if we look at many common diseases of civilization such as asthma, arthritis, cancer, eczema, migraine headaches and many others, there are many drugs that treat the symptoms but modern health care really does not have a concrete cure for them. If we always remember to try to find the core of the problem or the cause rather than dealing with a disease and symptoms, we will have greater success in solving the mysteries of our health. Treating the whole person through holistic methods such as Bowen therapy rather than just treating the disease is much more effective.

Special conditions and use of Bowen therapy:

There are a few special conditions where Bowen therapy has been very beneficial and are worthwhile noting.

Bowen therapy and children

The Bowen method can be extremely effective when used on children. I have used it for cases of eczema, asthma, hyper-activity, low immunity, bronchitis, ear infections, bedwetting and many other health problems with great success. Some young children may find it hard to stay still initially while on the massage table but after a few minutes usually calm down.

Bowen therapy and pregnancy

During pregnancy there are remarkable changes that occur and are times when problems may occur which can include back pain, morning sickness and other symptoms. Some applications of the Bowen method can even be used every day during this time especially for lower back pain, as changes are occurring daily in the pregnant woman. Bowen therapy has also been used effectively during labor.

Bowen therapy and the elderly

Since massage and other more aggressive methods can sometimes be painful or may even cause bruising or even injury to elderly clients, the gentle touch of the Bowen method is ideal for this kind of client. As we also mentioned early in this book, the healing ability of touch in the form of Bowen therapy is very therapeutic for the aging population and can assist in cases of depression, grief, loss of spouse and loneliness as well as many chronic health problems.

Bowen therapy and animals

The Bowen method has been used on many animals including cats, dogs and horses. There are now many established schools that teach the Bowen method on horses, as there is a great demand for methods to assist in injuries especially for the racehorse industry.

Bowen therapy, cancer and terminal illness

Many forms of massage are not recommended for cancer patients but the Bowen method can be used in most cases. It can be used for relief after chemotherapy or radiation therapy and is very beneficial in dealing with the stress of living with such a serious disease. The benefits of touch especially for those that are terminally ill become very significant during this time. I honestly believe that the power and gentle touch provided by Bowen therapy can provide soothing relief for the mind and body even during the last days of life.

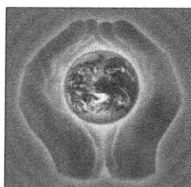

What patients have said after their Bowen session

During my many years of performing Bowen therapy on thousands of patients, I have heard so many reactions and comments after people have undergone this method. As these reactions varied so much from individual to individual and often were very surprising, a few years ago I began to start writing them down.

Often on their first visit, my patients have asked me, how will you feel after a series of Bowen sessions? I can never really say what reaction there will be to Bowen therapy as each client is different, nor can I ever promise any specific results. In some cases, the Bowen method has resulted in no significant improvements. However, in my experience and in over 80 percent of my cases, I have seen positive results.

Here is just a small sample of the thousands of responses or comments that I have had the remarkable privilege to hear over the years.

"I feel lighter, almost like I have had a few drinks."

"I have never been able to express my feelings with my husband and talk about our problems. The day after my Bowen session I told my husband really how I feel."

"The first day after my Bowen session, my pain completely disappeared, then the next day I felt like a truck had run over me. A few days later I started to feel much better."

"I used to have one migraine headache every week. After only 3 Bowen sessions, my migraine headaches disappeared com-

pletely for 6 months. They only come back occasionally now and are much less intense."

"I suffer from asthma and often have to use a bronchial dilator spray. After a few Bowen sessions, at first I had some heavy coughing fits, but afterwards it seemed that my breathing cleared up and I could breathe a lot easier."

"I suffered from pre-menstrual syndrome and irregular periods. After Bowen therapy, these monthly symptoms disappeared."

"I was barely able to walk up a set of stairs before I began my Bowen sessions. Now, all pain is gone and I have no problem climbing up several flights of stairs."

"I was scheduled for knee surgery for a sporting injury. After several Bowen sessions, the swelling went down and the pain went away. I did not have to have the knee operated on."

"I was not able to have children and we had tried for a few years. I decided to try the Bowen method and after several sessions I was able to become pregnant and now my husband and I can have the family that we have dreamed about."

"I was an avid tennis-player until I injured my shoulder and could not even raise up my hand. It seemed that for over a year I had pain in my shoulder. After Bowen therapy, my shoulder was able to finally heal, the pain went away and I could return back to playing tennis."

"I was sexually abused as a child and never told anyone about what had happened. After the Bowen method, I finally felt comfortable enough to talk about it. I feel an incredible sense of relief."

"My immune system was down and I found that I suffered many bouts of the flu every year. I tried the Bowen method, my immunity improved and I get sick less often now."

"I feel like I could run a marathon right now."

"I work many hours at the computer and my neck was so bad that I had trouble turning it from side to side. The Bowen method completely cured my problem."

"I suffered from chronic constipation. After several sessions of the Bowen method and increasing my water intake, I did not need to take any laxatives any more."

"I had a cyst and after only 3 Bowen sessions it disappeared all by itself."

"Right now I feel like there is extreme warmth on some areas of my back."

"I feel a bit dizzy and tired after my first Bowen session."

"I didn't feel any different except that I slept better."

"My jaw used to make a clicking noise when I ate. After the Bowen method, the clicking stopped."

"My legs and feet would swell up all the time. I made an appointment for Bowen therapy and now it does not happen any more."

"My feet and hands would often feel very cold. The Bowen method seemed to improve my circulation and it seems much better now."

"I was suffering from an intense burning sensation from a urinary tract infection. The Bowen method relieved all the pain after the first session."

"I had a lump in my breast and decided to try the Bowen method. After a few weeks the lump disappeared."

"After the Bowen method, I noticed that my urine was much darker for a few days."

"I was under extreme stress and could not concentrate. After the first Bowen session, I felt an incredible sense of calmness and relaxation."

"I was 7 months pregnant and suffering from lower back pain. The Bowen method helped to reduce the pain."

"I was suffering from high blood pressure. After several sessions of the Bowen method, my blood pressure dropped."

"I had recurrent bouts of eczema. I tried the Bowen method, at first the eczema became worse, but after several more sessions it cleared up and has not come back."

"I did not notice any difference after undergoing Bowen therapy, only that I felt a bit more relaxed."

"I was suffering from tinnitus or ringing in the ears. It was getting so bad that I could not sleep at night. After three sessions of the Bowen method, the ringing stopped and only occasionally comes back now."

"I was suffering from a slightly raised fever for a few months. The Bowen method helped it to go away."

"I feel much more calmer and in control after undergoing Bowen therapy."

"My 7 year old child was very hyperactive and was not concentrating at school. I made an appointment for him for a Bowen session and after a few weeks, he calmed down and started doing a lot better at school."

"After the divorce, my youngest daughter seemed to suffer psychologically. The Bowen method helped her to reduce the stress and anger she had within."

"I was suffering from digestive problems and stomach pain. I tried Bowen therapy for a few sessions, and it feels much better now."

"My joints and arthritis were causing me intense pain. I tried the Bowen method and I feel that my condition has dramatically improved and I have reduced my anti-inflammatory medication and pain medication."

"I suffer from chronic bronchitis. I made an appointment for the Bowen method and found that the wheezing that I suffered from improved dramatically."

"I was suffering from hot flushes during menopause and the Bowen method reduced their intensity."

"I had a tumor and after several sessions of the Bowen method, the doctors found that it had dramatically reduced in size."

"The next day after my Bowen session, I felt an incredible need to cry."

"I feel like an incredible weight has just lifted off of me."

"I was suffering from anxiety attacks. The Bowen method helped me to overcome them."

"My range of motion in my shoulder has improved significantly after the Bowen method."

"I was diagnosed with breast cancer and was experiencing a lot of stress. The Bowen method helped me to stop feeling sorry for myself and to keep a positive outlook on life."

"I was suffering from diabetes Type II, and the Bowen method helped me to stabilize my blood sugar levels."

"I found that my eyesight improved after the Bowen method."

"After my divorce, I felt that I was losing control of my life. I made an appointment for a Bowen therapy session and it has helped me to deal with the pain of the divorce."

"I had a lump under my arm for a long time. After Bowen therapy it disappeared."

"I was a heavy smoker and after my first Bowen session I started to cough up phlegm in large amounts, but afterwards my breathing improved."

"I was suffering from "tennis elbow" but it was completely healed after a few sessions of the Bowen method."

"I had suffered an ankle sprain and my ankle was swelled up. After one Bowen session, the swelling subsided and it healed very quickly afterwards."

"I was feeling extremely tired all the time. I came for a few Bowen sessions and much to my surprise my energy levels increased."

"I had constant stomach cramps and the pain disappeared immediately after the first Bowen session."

"Every spring I would suffer from hay fever but after a few Bowen sessions, the allergic reactions subsided."

"I feel tingling sensations in my legs and arms."

"During my Bowen session, I felt a sudden overwhelming feeling that came over me and I started to cry uncontrollably."

"When you apply the Bowen moves, I feel impulses traveling up and down my back and legs."

"As a child I had a knee injury. After the first Bowen session, I started to feel pain in my knee that I had not felt since the injury over 15 years ago. After a couple days the pain disappeared."

"I was suffering from Carpal Tunnel Syndrome and decided to try the Bowen method. After a few sessions the pain went away and I did not need to seek any further medical attention."

"I had a toothache and the pain immediately subsided after a Bowen session."

"The Bowen method has helped me to deal with my depression."

"Some moves that were administered felt very sensitive when I had my first Bowen session."

"I was suffering form insomnia probably due to a lot of stress at work. The first night after my Bowen therapy session I slept like a baby."

"The Bowen method helped reduce the pain from my varicose veins and improved my circulation."

"I found that I would often feel dizzy and sometimes would faint. The Bowen method helped me to improve my circulation and it does not happen any more."

"Right after my first Bowen session, I could not do anything but sleep. I felt very, very tired."

"I was not able to work out a problem I had, but after my Bowen session, I found I could think much more clearly and I solved the problem right away."

"It is hard to believe that such a gentle method could completely rid me of the pain that I have suffered from for years."

BOWEN THERAPY

Tom Bowen's gift to the world

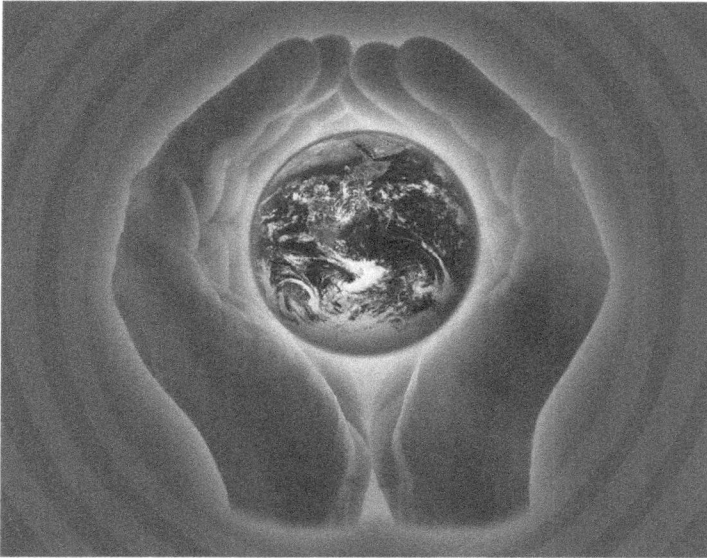

Conclusion:

A purely natural phenomenon

Conclusion:

Bowen Therapy - a purely natural phenomenon

Our society is often guilty of complicating our health care system as seen by the host of expensive diagnostic machines, chemical drugs and treatment methods not to mention the endless list of unnecessary operations that are performed year after year. The financial costs are enormous, not just the cost to health care but also the costs of side effects to patients. Unfortunately, these futile methods often fail as they do not address the cause of the problem or treat the person as a whole. The human being is not a machine or an experimental guinea pig. The human being is complex and that is why the future of medicine cannot center just on chemical drugs that treat only the symptoms of what is really happening inside. The future success of medicine is dependent on methods that will view the human being as a whole and consider all aspects that affect health status. While Bowen therapy is obviously not the answer to every health problem, I do believe that it is one important component of what I call holistic health care. Our body is an instrument of nature and we need to learn to treat it as such.

Bowen therapy is truly a purely natural phenomenon. Its use requires no needles, no sophisticated machines, heating pads or electricity, just a series of gentle moves that abide by the laws of nature. Perhaps that is why it is so effective and why the body responds in so many amazing ways.

In all my years working with natural medicine I have never come across a more effective and pain-free body therapy technique, as is the Bowen method. Today it is taught in over 25 countries and used by doctors, physiotherapists, chiropractors, massage therapists, nurses and other health professionals across the globe. Every year its popularity grows due to its very high success rate and universal application for a diverse list of health conditions.

Tom Bowen certainly knew what he was doing back in Geelong, Australia many years ago. He was ahead of his time. He was a true pioneer of nature's ability to cure. He knew then that the secrets to health did not come in a pill bottle but in learning how to stimulate the body so that it could activate its own healing powers. The Bowen community owes a lot to this dedicated man as do the thousands and thousands of people whose health problems have been assisted by his method.

Even after so many Bowen sessions that I have performed on so many clients, I am still to this day in awe of what the method can sometimes achieve. I still can't help feeling surprised whenever a migraine headache stops, when chronic back pain disappears, when clients report feelings of increased energy, euphoria and heightened awareness. It fills me with great hope that perhaps someday we can tackle our health problems in a completely different way than we have in the past. Perhaps we will one day learn to respect the human body and to listen to its natural needs. As I have mentioned before, we are only at the tip of the iceberg of what we know. What other secrets will we uncover about the human mind, body and spirit? It brings me great joy to have had the privilege to follow that fleeting mist in the fog that appeared to me many years ago, to decide to learn the Bowen method and to have the opportunity to help so many people because of it and to now pass it on to others. Every reaction and life process that goes on inside of us is really quite a miracle and every Bowen move and what it triggers in the body is a miracle in itself. With every success it always serves to remind me that there are forces within the body that we are just starting to understand. Modern medicine may never quantify these forces or scientifically explain them, but I am sure Tom Bowen is up there somewhere smiling down on all of us, not at all surprised at how it has helped so many.

Just as Mr. Bowen will always be remembered as a great pioneer of natural medicine, we are each in our own way pioneers each time we decide to find an alternative way to deal with our health problems, especially methods that do not include chemical drugs. As his method grows along with other natural drug-free methods of dealing with disease, the foundation is set for new pioneers to emerge as we slowly uncover the magical secrets of holistic human health. Those who have been touched by the magic of Bowen therapy as I have, cannot help but move one step closer to reinforcing the belief that by abiding to nature's laws we can truly achieve the optimum health that we all deserve. The harmony of the human mind, body and spirit in symbiosis with the environment around us, is quite simply, the greatest natural phenomenon of all.

Wishing you the best of natural holistic health,

Frank Navratil BSc. N.D.

RETURN TO HEALTH ®

OTHER BOOKS BY FRANK NAVRATIL, BSC. N.D.

If you have enjoyed this book by Frank Navratil BSc. N.D., read these books also by the same author:

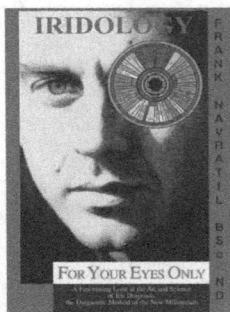

IRIDOLOGY – FOR YOUR EYES ONLY

Iridology is an art and a science that allows one to diagnose the physical and psychological health status of an individual by signs in the pupil, iris, and sclera of the eye. This book shares the results of extensive studies of thousands of eyes by Frank Navratil BSc. N.D., a world-renowned iridologist, naturopath and clinical nutritionist.

Frank Navratil BSc. N.D. presents his fascinating experiences with natural medicine and iridology that will open your eyes and mind to a new view on health and medicine.

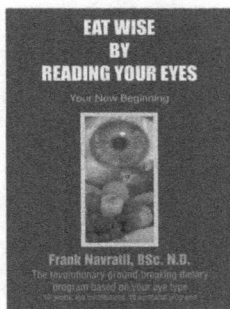

EAT WISE BY READING YOUR EYES

Your New Beginning

The revolutionary ground - breaking dietary program based on your eye type

This unique, easy to follow nutritional program uses genetic make-up based on eye-type so that you can:

· Maintain ideal body weight
· Stay physically and mentally healthy
· Prevent or cure disease

(For a lifetime)

HOLISTIC HEALING CARDS

A set of full color cards and comprehensive handbook that teach the basis of holistic or whole health: the harmony of the mind, body and spirit using nature's healing methods. These 40 cards and handbook, written and designed by Frank Navratil, BSc. N.D. are full of inspirational messages and explain how you can uncap your powers of intuition and enlighten your understanding of your holistic healing needs. Use these cards whenever you feel low in energy, depressed, unbalanced, lost, anxious or confused, when sick, when desiring answers to chronic health problems or when seeking answers for a friend or loved one.

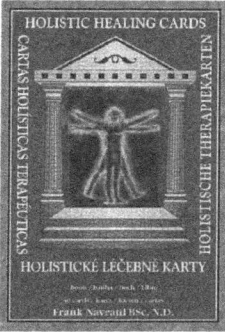

Others soon to come...

To order:
e-mail: irisproducts@irisdiagnosis.org
www.irisdiagnosis.org

Return to Health International

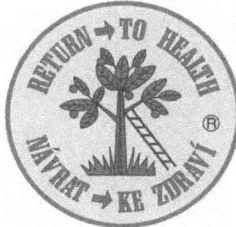

Welcome to the world of natural medicine

RETURN TO HEALTH ®

NATURAL MEDICINE COURSES ON CD-ROM BY FRANK NAVRATIL, BSC. N.D.

Please contact us if you are interested in taking any of these exciting courses written by Frank Navratil BSc. N.D. about nutritional health and natural medicine.

Holistic Nutrition Courses on CD-ROM

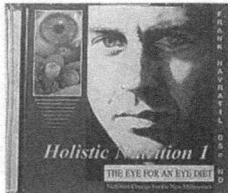

Holistic Nutrition 1

Holistic Nutrition 2

Holistic Nutrition 3

www.irisdiagnosis.org

Return to Health International College of Natural Medicine

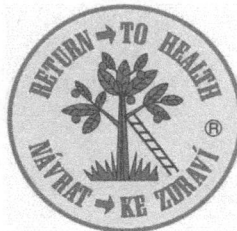

Welcome to the world of natural medicine

RETURN TO HEALTH ®

NATURAL MEDICINE COURSES ON CD-ROM BY FRANK NAVRATIL, BSC. N.D.

Iridology Courses on CD-ROM

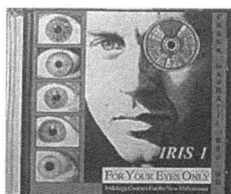

Iris 1 - Beginner Iridology

Iris 2 - Intermediate Iridology

Iris 3 - Advanced Iridology

Contact

To order iridology and holistic nutrition books and products
or for information on our CD-ROM home study courses contact us at:
e-mail: irisproducts@irisdiagnosis.org

www.irisdiagnosis.org

Return to Health International College of Natural Medicine

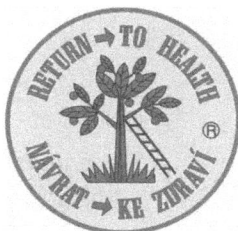

Welcome to the world of natural medicine

INDEX

ABOUT THE AUTHOR

Frank Navratil, BSc. N.D. was born of Czech parents in Vancouver, Canada. He studied physiology and nutrition in university. During the 90's he moved to Sydney, Australia where he studied alternative medicine, iridology and the Bowen method and practiced as a naturopath, iridologist, Bowen therapist and clinical nutritionist. From 1997, he lives in Prague where he currently runs a successful naturopathic practice, lectures around the world and is the director of an international school that offers a variety of courses in natural medicine. He is a world-renowned iridologist and many doctors and therapists around the world have used his methods of iridology and nutrition.

In the Czech Republic, Australia, Europe, the United States and many other countries, he has lectured on the theme of iridology and nutrition and has appeared on many television and radio programs centered on natural means of diagnosis and holistic healing. Many of his books have been translated into several other languages.

His practice and beliefs focus on natural holistic methods that allow the body to heal itself. These include iridology, vitamin and mineral therapy, Bowen therapy, nutrition and diet and lifestyle changes.

Printed in August 2023
by Rotomail Italia S.p.A., Vignate (MI) - Italy